PODIATRY BUSINESS SUCCESS SECRETS

The Ultimate Guide to Building a Profitable Podiatry Practice

That Works Without You

Lorcan O Donaile, *Podiatrist & Health Business Mentor*

To Paola,

www.morepracticeprofits.com

Hope you enjoy the book!
Best Wishes,
Lorcan

Copyright © 2020 by Lorcan O Donaile

ISBN: 9781655040580

DEDICATION

I want to dedicate this book to long suffering wife Sinead who has stood by me and always told me I could do it even when I doubted myself.

I also want to dedicate it to all those Podiatrists who roll the dice and have the courage to set out on their own.
I know the tenacity it takes and I salute you.

DOWNLOAD THE BONUSES AVAILABLE FOR READERS OF THIS BOOK FOR FREE AT ...

www.morepracticeprofits.com/podiatry-business-book-bonus

Just to say thanks for reading my book, I would like to give you lots of FREE resources you can use today in your clinic to help you

Earn More, Work Less & Enjoy Life

Contents

Start Here...7

Secret No 1. Great Clinical Skills Will Not Guarantee A Profitable Podiatry Practice 17

Secret No 2. You Need A Business Mindset.......................................31

Secret No 3. You Need To Wow Them With Your Customer Service ..43

Secret No 4. Fix Your Leaky Bucket First...55

Secret No 5. You Need A Robust Price Strategy 71

Secret No 6. You Have Got To Know Your Numbers. 81

Secret No 7. Why Almost All Podiatry Clinics Are Wasting Their Money On Marketing..95

Secret No 8.. Always Use The Marketing Triad. 111

Secret No 9. Start With Internal Marketing, It's Simpler By Far...........125

Secret No 10. Rock Your Podiatry Clinic With Amazing External Marketing...141

Secret No 11. Staff, You Have To Learn To Love Them. 179

Secret No 12. How do I scale my podiatry clinic?.............................201

Secret No 13. Get A Podiatry Business Coach................................211

About The Author...217

Start Here...

I heard a statistic recently that the dropout rate in my profession, Podiatry, in Ireland where I live and the UK where I trained back in the day is somewhere near 50% over 10 years from the time that podiatrists qualify. Now, I don't know if this is still correct, or a slight exaggeration, but I do know anecdotally that there does seem to be quite a large dropout rate, certainly in podiatry and I suspect also in similar professions or medical services like physiotherapy.

Why does this happen?

I think this is happening for two reasons. The first is the job is not what they expected and they then have two options, they can move into the health service which can be quite a frustrating place to work. The Health Service here in Ireland and the NHS in the UK, is completely free for patient's and that's brilliant. You cannot necessarily see the patient as often as you might like to do and you've often got to rush that appointment as the case load is so large.

For a lot of clinicians who are independent minded, they feel hamstrung in their ability to progress within the confines of the service and its associated bureaucracy and thus the ability to comprehensively help those patients.

Secondly, the other option is to move into private practice. This can seem quite daunting. When they look around at other practitioners working in private practice including physiotherapy, podiatry, and so forth, they appear to be doing long hours and have little or no real pay security. Quite a lot of them seem to be quite stressed and don't have the reassurance of the public sector pension or holiday pay.

Why would they give up a job with a pension and a secure wage every week to move into private practice? Indeed, why do people do this at all? I believe they do so because they hope that there is a better way to be fulfilled in their profession. Many clinic owners feel that by plowing their own furrow they can deliver best practice medical care and still provide themselves with financial independence and a better quality of life that they yearn for.

This is why they roll the dice, take out that loan, leave that job and open those doors. To those of you thinking of opening your own clinic or have already done so let me say at this point, congratulations, you are the few, the less than 5% of the world's population that will ever do so. It takes great courage to start your own business. The reality of private practice ownership is it can be a tough and lonely enterprise.

I know of a medic who had been 40 years building his business, and at the end of it couldn't find anyone to take it over and couldn't sell it. Instead, he had to close it down and just rent the rooms. 85% of small businesses never sell.

Why is this?

I believe it's because they're not true businesses.

What they really are is a job. Sometimes they are a well paid job, but a job all the same where the owner cannot leave the business for any protracted period of time because the business is wholly dependent on them. This was me a number of years ago. Things don't have to be this way though.

At this point, you're probably not sure what a health business coach will do for you. That's fair enough. When I first heard of the idea of a business coach for my clinic I was very unsure if that was right for me. I didn't want it to be commercialized or sold to or worse made into some sleazy sales person doing unethical things in my clinic just to make a quick buck.

Let's face it, when we go through university, getting our degree pretty much all the emphasis is on us getting to a basic level of clinical competence. During my term time in University in London, I got one hour of business training on how to run a private practice. It was given by one of the only podiatrists who worked in the clinic who also owned a private practice.

I assume he was chosen because he was wore the sharpest suit and seemed to believe he knew what he was doing. When I look back now, I know that he didn't.

When I started my own clinic seven years later, I was really clueless on what it took to run a successful podiatry clinic. I'd spent a month doing a 25 page business plan that none of the banks I met bothered to read. I still have it and I take it out every once in a while to remind myself how far I've come.

I know I am not alone. As medical professionals, we are really well trained and know how to be thorough in patient care, devise a diagnosis of the problems, work out a solution and see the plan through to the end. However when it comes to the business side, we are not at all sure about how to do the same thing.

How do we transfer our clinical skills into enough income to allow us to reach the personal and professional goals we vaguely talked about when we give up our paid job to open our own clinic?

Maybe we are making good money and delivering a really good service but the clinic is too dependent on us, meaning we are tied to the clinic. It dawns on us after a while that really what we have built for ourselves is a really well paid job rather than a proper standalone business.

Well, this is where a health business coach will come in. They look at your business from a distance and see the opportunities as well as the problems.

Of course your business has some problems. You're not likely to be reading this if everything was perfect and you reckon, naturally, that any health business coach worth their salt will be able to spot those problems.

A Health Business Coach should, with you, come up with a plan to work through these problems and as a business coach will also be detached enough from your clinic they will be able to spot the low hanging fruit or opportunities to get quick wins.

It's not all about spending lots of money on marketing or getting into the hippest social media craze. Often there is plenty that can be achieved with what you already have before spending any extra money on marketing.

I spent 18 months looking at the opportunities inside my own clinic, doubling my profits for no extra spend before turning to paid marketing.

Health business coach will keep you accountable.

Having someone you are paying to check up on you and your business is a sure fire way to ensure effective steps are implemented. Having a Business Coach that you check in with regularly means that you know there is a deadline to get the work you agreed done, delivered on time.

Us humans are all the same. We will leave it off until tomorrow if we can go off the after shiny objects instead. Just ask my wife what am I like fixing things around the house. Knowing you have a call coming will mean you can't put off the important stuff that will be needed to get your business into shape.

A health business coach gives you focus so you get the best results from the least effort. All clinic owners are busy. It can be a real juggling act trying to treat patients handle staff, accounts, bills, marketing and day to day running of the clinic. Family is usually the first thing to get jettisoned. A good coach will show you that you can't do it all yourself, teach you what to focus on to get the best bang for your buck and what to delegate.

A decent Health Business Coach knows what it takes to turn your clinic into a passive business. At one point I was working well over 40 hours a week treating patients doing accounts, wages etc in evenings and weekends and even making my own insoles in a workshop up to 11pm at night.

No matter how hard I worked, I still couldn't afford to slow down as the clinic depended on the income I generated so much. When my wife came home with our first child, I took only six hours off. Time I'll never get back.

I now do four hours clinical a week because I choose to, take four holidays a year away from the business and it runs fine without me with my patients still getting the same quality clinical care. Last summer, I took all of August off logged in twice remotely for 40 minutes to see how things were going and came back to a clinic that had had its highest ever monthly turnover.

I now have a true business that delivers exceptional customer service and best practice patient care by a well trained team that don't need me there every day to keep things running.

One of my favorite clients, let's just call him john doe, contacted me initially, because he was having problems with his clinic. On the outside, he looked like he had a very successful clinic he'd been open for over 10 years and seemed quite happy and jolly.

However this was not the truth. When he reached out to me, he was stressed both financially and emotionally. He couldn't take a holiday for more than seven days because he needed the cash flow to keep the clinic running. He was at breaking point and considering closing up altogether and going back to a secure NHS job.

After about three months, I remember him saying to me on one of our calls, "For the first time in years, I feel in charge of my own business." He could see the future. He could see what was possible, and that he would get to the point where he had a true business that provided him with the income he desired to live the life he wanted and make a choice on how hard and how often he would see patient's.

When it boils down to it, what most clinic owners really want is to feel fulfilled.

Money is important, but it is not everything.

What most clinical owners really want is a clinic that gives them enough money to make it worth the hassle.

A clinic that's not so dependent on them that they are tied to it all of the time.

They want a business that delivers them freedom to choose.

That is what a health business coach will do for you. I help my clients develop the type of business that delivers you the freedom you choose and reach your life goals.

Whether we ever meet or not my sincere wish for you reading this book is that you start the journey towards moving from a clinic to a true business that still provides best practice medical care, exceptional customer service, and allows you to earn more, work less and live your life to the full.

This book can be read by reading any chapter you wish at a time. However, I recommend you read it in the order it's written. In all likelihood you will want to go straight to the marketing sections to see how do I get more patients because that's the answer isn't it.....

"I just more patient's, don't I" ?

The truth is it's not the answer. Not the first answer anyway.

Good luck. I hope you enjoy the book

Lorcan Ó Donaile, *Podiatrist & Podiatry & Health Business Mentor*

www.morepracticeprofits.com

SECRET NO 1.

Great Clinical Skills Will Not Guarantee A Profitable Podiatry Practice

So, why did I write this book?

I wrote this book for you, the clinic owner or potential clinic owner.

Yes I am a podiatrist, but whether you are a Podiatrist, Physiotherapist, Osteopath, Chiropractor, Speech Therapist, Occupational Therapist, etc. and if you're either thinking about opening your own clinic or have already done so, then this book is 100% for you.

Obviously I'm a podiatrist and it's written from a podiatrist perspective, but the concepts I talk about throughout this book can be transferred to any sort of health professionals clinic.

I got up every morning for longer than I wanted to at 5 am to type some more words in the hope that I could help you avoid the mistakes I made. Mistakes that meant that I only took one foreign holiday in the first 10 years of opening my business. Mistakes that meant that I never had enough to buy a home or get a pension for longer than that.

Mistakes that made me question why I ever chose the path I did. Why didn't I do something else altogether in college?

I wrote this book to show you that there is another way, a way that means that you do not have to be the first to arrive if you own your own clinic and the last to leave.

I wrote this book to show you that you do not have to be the last to get paid, to show you that you don't have to be tied to that clinic forever.

You can pick and choose when you want to want to see patients, and yet still make a good income and provide you and your loved ones with the lifestyle you seek.

When I first started my clinic I assumed that all I needed to do was to be good at clinical work and as I was good at clinical work my lifestyle would be rewarded.

This was not the case.

It took me a long time to realise that patients don't really care how well qualified you are or how many courses you've gone on. They really don't care whether you've done your CPD or not.

Now I'm not saying you shouldn't do these things, but to patient's they're not really that interested.

Why should they care?

All they really care about is can you help them get them better and are you going to deliver on that promise of getting them better.

It took me a long time to realise that customer service, pricing, key performance indicators(KPI's), knowing your numbers, marketing (both internal and external) and how to handle staff were all necessary for me to be able to scale up my business to the point where I didn't need to work there all of the time.

I could still earn more, work less and provide an even better quality service to my patients for longer hours, than happened when I was on my own.

I wish I had read a book like this when I first started my clinic or even three or four years in but the kind of I wanted to read,a book like this for podiatrists in particular, did not exist.

So when I set up my Podiatry Business Mentorship programme I promised myself that I would write the kind of book I would have wanted to read.

Before I get on to the rest of the book I want to just tell you a little about my journey so you can see that I too have been in the trenches of owning and running a small clinic with little or no profit and have overcome these difficulties. You can do it too. I should know.... I have. Here's how....

My Story.

I grew up in the countryside, on the west coast of Ireland with two older brothers and two older sisters. When I came to finishing my secondary level education I wasn't too sure what I wanted to do. I ended up drifting into podiatry as my brother in law was a podiatrist as I liked the idea of doing something to do with science and I wanted to be able to finish work at five o'clock. Saying I was naive would be an understatement.

When I was 18 I moved to London & I went to college in London Foot Hospital and University College London. I completed a degree and Podiatric Medicine and qualified in 1998.

Back then, there weren't too many jobs for podiatrists in Ireland and I wanted to move home. My brother in law offered me a job as he was getting very busy and wanted to expand his clinic. I took the position and worked for him for seven years. I learned a lot in that clinic, but felt a lot of frustration at the same time, especially in the final years. This is no fault of his but more mine, my personality is one where I don't like to be told what to do.

My wife says I'm very stubborn. She's probably right, in fact I know she's right. I was offered a partnership in the clinic, but decided instead that I needed to leave. I wanted to set out on my own path and felt as the clinic I was working in had all of that money coming in that if I could do that then when opened my own clinic it would surely be fine except i would get to keep the profits for myself. Like I said I was very naive.

This is what most of us new comers do. We work for someone else and then we think well I can do all the clinical work, why not keep all the money. So we open a clinic. And after a number of years we realise it's not as simple as that.

The money's coming in but just as quickly it's going out. In some cases it's going out faster than it's coming in. We run out of cash flow and we close the clinic.

Anyway I quit my full time job having been offered a partnership. My parents thought I was crazy. I decided to convince my then girlfriend, now wife, to quit her full time pensionable job too and we both went travelling.

I don't regret this. I would hate to be nearing retirement haven't been afraid to take the chance. Even knowing the stress and trauma that was to follow I would still do it again but with some changes to how I did it of course.

After six months travelling and running up a bit of debt I came back home and moved to Cork city on the south coast of Ireland. I decided to write a business plan and this took about a month to do as I was doing what all the books say to do. To say the business plan was a waste of time wouldn't be quite fair, but it wasn't a lot of help either and I now take it out every once in a while for the laugh.

I opened the doors in 2005, and grew to capacity within about 18 to 24 months. I was flat out so I took on a part time receptionist to begin with, but I had no idea how to train her really.

I was running a typical one clinician business.

It was all on me.

I had no wages if I took a holiday.

I never took a holiday beyond seven days.

I worked really long hours. It was not unusual for me to work 60 to 70 hours a week.

I never knew my numbers.

For example with regards to tax I had zero planning in place. I would get a tax bill in September due in October for the

Calendar year before and have to figure out in a rush how to pay it.

I freely admit, I had no clue what I was doing in regards to the business.

I was good clinically. I was getting really good clinical outcomes and patients were happy. This is why I had grown the clinic so fast.

There seemed to be a lot of money coming in. But there was never enough. Not enough to pay the wages or to make the receptionist go full time. Never enough to pay the rent, and still have some left over for me to live off, and to try and build a life.

I really didn't know my numbers, and I was living beyond my means as a result. Like most business owners, I was afraid to know the truth, and I never really questioned my accountant. I was afraid to know what he would say.

This went on for about eight to nine years. I was really stressed out with anxiety my constant companion and didn't know what I to do to get myself out of the hole I found myself in.

By lucky chance I used to listen to a lot of podcasts and one time I heard a podcast about a running a healthcare business and heard mention of a book, a business book about scaling up your business called the E-myth by Michael Gerber. I quickly bought the book on Amazon and decided, having read it that I would scale up.

However, what I would do is do it on the cheap, doing it all by myself to avoid the cost of a mentor. This was a huge mistake, but understandable as I couldn't justify to myself spending more money on a mentor, when I already didn't have enough money.

Again, not knowing what I was doing I took on a physiotherapist and followed this with another podiatrist and paid them a percentage of wage, another huge mistake.

I did some marketing, well basically I did whatever marketing someone came in and asked me to buy, but I was not sure what I was doing.

Again, I didn't want to spend any money on some professional help, so did it all myself.

I never measured my outcomes and I had no idea how successful or otherwise my marketing was, just like most clinic owners I meet now. When I was asked, what was marketing like I would say it was nearly all word of mouth, meaning I didn't have any marketing, or I didn't know how I got new patients.

To the outsider it looked great. I had five staff, I was able to take an unpaid holiday every year. I seem to have a successful business. I was all smiles. But inside, I was crumbling.

By now wife was questioning why we'd ever done this to begin with and I had at this point three children that depended on me with no sign of us ever being able to buy a house even with a drop in house prices of 33% during that time in Ireland. I was living with a non secure tenancy and stresses were building and building.

At one point I came back from a holiday with my family to find a staff threatening me with employer tribunal because I did not know my responsibilities. When I look back on it now I realise that I was completely clueless and deserving of their wrath.

I was extremely anxious all of the time and in big trouble financially. I had a big lease I couldn't afford and I couldn't afford to scale a business any further, because I couldn't afford the wages. I had a large tax bill, bigger even than my entire years profit and no way to pay it.

As I didn't know what I was doing and when it came to my accounts, banks would not help me and I was facing down a tax audit. I would regularly go to sleep wondering how I was going to pay the wages and the tax that week.

I was the worst paid in the clinic and for 4 Christmases in a row, did not pay myself any wage as the clinic was closed. There was inconsistent cash flow and I couldn't afford to pay myself and the staff therefore, the staff got paid first.

This also affected my marriage, as I was extremely stressed and my home life was poor due to my mood swings. I have a very patient wife. I remember driving home from work on Friday crying, wishing I could crawl into bed and not have to wake up again, as it couldn't face what I had to deal with the following week.

How did I arrive at this place I asked myself?

I had thought all I needed was Clinical Excellence and I did not want to pay for any help as I was so broke.

Obviously as you're reading this book you realise that things did change. But how did I change things around?

Well I am very stubborn. I admit it freely. I wouldn't give in. I decided I was going to have to get some help, no matter how broke I was. I got some really good help including changing my accountant who went into forensic detail with my living expenses and costs associated with the business.

I paid for a business coach and business mentoring expert help and decided I would apply the same approach as I would in clinical learning to my business.

What I mean by this is we clinicians are trained to do best medical practice using research and to apply that best practice and research in our clinical reasoning. I used this process in my business.

I read everything I could that was relevant.

I studied.

I attended courses.

I listened to experts, and I was willing to pay for this education and help just like I would be willing to pay a good quality Podiatry CPD course up until then.

I continue to do this throughout my career. And as I write this still have two paid mentors that I talked to every single month.

Don't let me pretend that this was easy. It was not easy. This was the hardest thing I've done in a long, long time.

But it has paid off.

I now have a clinic, a true business, that provides 500% more treatments to patients than it did when I worked on my own.

My profits have gone up 400% and are still climbing and I personally can pick and choose who I want to treat and when I'm available to do so.

Right now, I treat patients for 4- 5 hours a week and I am in the clinic for approximately two hours per day, and spend the rest of my time educating other clinic owners, on how to do the same in their clinic.

I show them how to get out of the position where you can't afford to take a break, because the clinic is depending on you.

I show them how to earn more, work less and start to live your life.

When you first begin this journey to improving your clinic and your quality of life it can seem like a mammoth task.

One of my favourite sayings is how to eat an elephant? One bite at a time.

It's a process. One step at a time working through the system. Over time, we change your clinic into a business that is relatively independent of you and that will continue to provide you with an income, whether you're there or not.

You can do this and make sure your clinic still provides the same excellent quality customer service and clinical outcomes to your patients as it would if you were seeing them yourself.

I've broken this book down into a number of chapters including mindset, customer service, Key Performance Indicators(KPI's) and marketing.

Now I know we all want to jump straight into the marketing, because we think the answer is just more patients, but it's not.

Take your time, go through the basics.

When a patient comes into you, you don't start treating them straight away. First you do your subjective, then you do your objective. It's the same with this process.

You need to know how your business is functioning from day to day first. Where is the low hanging fruit first.

The secret to having a podiatry clinic that allows you to grow a great team and delivers a great service even when you are on holiday is realising that having great clinical skills is simply not enough, you need great business skills too.

SECRET NO 2.

You Need A Business Mindset

The very first thing I work on with my private coaching clients is their mindset. The correct mindset is the key to unlocking a profitable clinic that delivers for both you, your staff, your patients and your suppliers.

We medical clinicians been conditioned to work in the health service. This is certainly true with regard to Podiatrists. Our role is to help patients with their health, which is admirable and is the whole purpose of our career and life long education.

However public health services often train us to treat that patient as quickly as possible and get them back out the door as we have a list of other patients waiting in the waiting room. We get no training on how to run a profitable business or how to charge patient's money for the services we provide.

Indeed I have met many public service based clinicians who suggest that we shouldn't be charging patients at all as money is an evil in medicine. Often Medical clinicians, having gone 3, 4 or 5 years through college will get their qualifications believing that it's immoral, or unethical to take money off of our patient's. Yet somehow we expect to run a business, pay for our lifestyle, our staff and our suppliers without taking enough money from patient's to make this happen.

We are extremely uncomfortable with asking patients for payments at the end of treatment, and we have no idea how to set our prices. Often we look around the locality, see what all the other clinics are charging and take an average price for fear or "charging too much". These same clinic owners never put their prices up, even though our costs are continually rising,citing that patient's in their area simply wouldn't pay anymore.

This University training, while excellent at on a clinical level is letting us down when it comes to actually making a profitable career outside of the health service were we would have the safety net of a wage every week and a pension. This is despite significant numbers of podiatrist working in private practice.

This is why we have such a high stress rate in the allied health professionals and a large dropout rate, certainly in my profession podiatry much higher than most would expect. Our education does not equip us to know how to handle staff or how to hold them accountable for their job.

Unbelievably we are often conditioned to believe that marketing is unethical. Indeed I remember going to a weekend

CPD course a number of years ago and sitting around a table with a bunch of physiotherapists, all of whom were in private practice and the general agreement among them all was that there was no need for a website that marketing was held in contempt.

"Why would I need to tell my patient what I do?" Patient's would just come to them by word of mouth.

I kept quiet but in my head I thought this was total bull. What use was an unprofitable clinic to anyone? What use is it to a patient coming in to see an overworked clinician who stressed out because of money, wages, not being able to take a holiday because every depending on them.

You are no longer just a clinician if you own your own clinic.

The key thing to know at this point to this is you need to get your mindset right first before you proceed any further in the journey of opening and owning your own profitable clinic.

If you either have your own clinic now or you're considering opening one you must remember that you are in business now. You are no longer just a clinician, you are no longer just that podiatrist,physiotherapist, osteopath that you were when you left college.

You are more than that now. Yes you are that clinician but you are also a business person. You are a marketer. You are a boss to your staff and you have responsibilities to all of those people.

What is the purpose of your business?

The purpose of your business is to provide you with the lifestyle that you want. Too often we leave a secure job working in another clinic or in the public health services thinking that when we open our own clinic we will be able to do things our way and make a great income too. Instead after a number of years we realise that we're stressed out, losing empathy for our patient's and it has just not turned out as we expected it would.

Let me repeat it again ... the purpose of your business is to provide you with the lifestyle that you set out to achieve when you opened your doors.

It also is there to provide your staff with the working environment where they are encouraged to be the best they can be and be protected by knowing that have a secure job. They need to know they work for an owner who's not stressed and is in charge of their destiny and the destiny of their business, allowing them to concentrate on providing for your patient's.

The purpose of your business is to provide for your patients and to make sure that they reached their goals and outcomes that they wish to achieve when they initially contact you. Over and over again I've met clinicians who feel that should only see the patient once or twice.

I would argue that by doing so, as it is unlikely that they have not fixed that chronic condition in one or two appointments that that patient has therefore wasted their money by coming to you in the first place, and will continue to do so as they move from clinic to clinic only having one two or three appointments and never getting 100% better.

The purpose of your business is to make sure that your suppliers are looked after that they don't have to wait for you to pay them. That you are not trying to dodge that next phone call from them because you haven't got the money to settle your bill.

All of this is your responsibility as the clinic owner. I know it's a lot to have on your shoulders, but this is what owning a business and running a profitable clinic is all about.

You have 2 options.

The way I see it, this can be done in two ways. It can be done the way that most clinics do it, which is following the University/Health Service model, where you work all the hours you can, you charge the same as your competitors and just keep your head above water. You carry on for 40 years and then you retire with very little. In almost all cases these clinic owners are unable to sell their business when the time comes as nobody wants to take on that lifestyle.

The alternative option is you change your mindset. You realise you are in business and that it is okay and ethical to do so. Millions of businesses around the world open their doors every single day and charge a price to ensure that they deliver a profit which in turn will deliver for the business owners, the business's staff, the business's customers and its suppliers.

Paradoxically, in most cases we look on this as perfectly normal and perfectly ethical yet when it comes to health care we seem to have a barrier to charging and believe that we should not charge our patient's *"too much"* or try and make a profit. Somehow we view it as immoral to make a decent profit.

The funny thing is your patients don't see it like this. Patients expect and indeed want you to make a profit. Otherwise you won't be open. You won't be there when they need you.

If I look at my own clinic for a moment. I used to work 40-50 hours a week, stressed out, couldn't take a holiday or a break. Since I changed my mindset my clinic is now open 500% more hours per week, allowing us to help even more patients while delivering a better quality service with less stress in the clinic.

We're open 12 hours a day, every day and Saturdays. This means our patients have the ability to come both before and after work and the extra profits allows us to invest in the latest technology and training, making sure that our patients get the best quality outcomes.

So, how do we work on mindset?

When I start working with a private client, in my coaching/ mentoring business the first thing we look at is their systems or their lack thereof. Most of us have these structures and systems in our clinic we just don't know we have them.

We've never written them down.

We've never thought about the fact that we have any systems.

An example is how we answer the phone. We tend to say the same thing over and over again. We just don't realise that we do so and perhaps if we sat down and thought about it we could improve it. I try to instil into my clients that these structures and systems if improved and implemented throughout the business would allow them to get their staff to provide the treatment and service that they would do themselves if they were treating that patient. This gives them free time to start to develop and work on the business itself.

The truly successful successful clinic owners, realise that they cannot see all patients all of the time. By implementing good quality structures good quality systems and training their staff on those systems and then holding them accountable to these systems are we able to scale up their business, see even more patients and give better quality care.

Like I said earlier, the purpose of your business is primarily to provide you the owner with the lifestyle that you wanted. If you look at your local shop owner down the road or the guy who owns the car garage or the newsagent next door you wouldn't expect him to go to work for free or at no profit.

It's a given that he's doing it to provide himself with the lifestyle that he wants. This can certainly be done ethically and there's no need to assume that doing so means you are trying to fleece your patient's. In Western society we understand that hard work, owning a business and all the stresses that go with it deserves to be rewarded.

Mindset is something that will continue to evolve for you as a business owner. When first I started to get to work with coaches for myself, my mindset was focused on simply having enough to pay the bills from week to week.

Now my mindset has changed to a point where I want to help other clinic owners who are struggling like I was. Hence I'm writing this book, and hence you are reading it.

So to begin, I'm going to give you some homework.

I want you to write out, and if you wish (in fact i would strongly recommend) show your significant other your answers.

Step 1;

Write out who do you like to be with most outside of work and why?

Life can't all the all about work. Personally, I like to spend time with my wife and kids. It gives me the most joy in my day.

Step 2;

What 3 things do you like to do most outside of work and how does it make you feel when you do these things?

Step 3;

What would it take to make you truly fulfilled personally?

I'm going to pause here and say to that I would recommend that you take your time at this even if it takes you a few days that's okay.

The answers to these 3 questions will change as you develop and get older and your life changes. That's okay too. The answers you have now don't have to be those that you keep for the rest of your life.

This is a process whereby you understand what your business is there for.

Step 4;

Once you have the answer to these and you know what you want out of life, then you work out how much money do you need to achieve these goals. Be as accurate as you can. Don't just throw a figure down on a piece of paper because this is important.

Step 5;

I then want you to write out what kind of business you would like to have and what you see yourself doing in the business in ...

A. 90 days,

B. 1 year,

C. 5 years and

D. What's your big, hairy, audacious goal.

Your big hairy audacious goal is a goal that you think you'd love to have if there were no limits to what you could do in your business. It doesn't mean you're going to get there but if you don't have a goal, how can you strive towards that goal.

I like to cycle, but I find if I haven't put my name down for a sportive I don't train half as hard and I don't get as much out of my cycling. Similarly by writing down you goals and working towards those goals you are far more likely to achieve those goals.

The purpose of all of this, is it let you know what you want your life to look like? What do you want your business to provide you with. Then you know what kind of business you need and how much you need financially to make, allowing you structure your business and your lifestyle around this.

You'd be surprised how many businesses out there never do this sort of stuff. They just go in every day. Park in the same place. Open the door. Do the same thing all day, every day ..... for 40 years.

It's no wonder 85% of small businesses, including small medical clinics, never sell. Wouldn't it be great when retirement comes along that you can sell on your business for a great price?

Once you have completed these steps, share these business goals with your significant other.

Indeed, send them on to me at info@morepracticeprofits. com .

If you're stuck or you're not sure how to do this drop me an email or connect with me on Facebook or Linkedin

So start the process of Earning More, Working Less & Living Life by working on your mindset and remember to keep doing so throughout your business life.

It's your responsibility to yourself, your staff, your patients your suppliers and most especially your family, that you build a business that provides you with the lifestyle that you want.

Didn't you quit that job and start your clinic to build a business that gives you the financial and personal freedom you desire?

The secret to having the podiatry clinic you always wanted is to have the right mindset.

The right mindset will ensure you begin to develop a clinic and business that delivers the financial and personal freedom we all want and ensures that your patients get the best quality care and achieve their health outcomes.

Isn't this exactly why you started to your clinic to begin with?

SECRET NO 3.

You Need To Wow Them With Your Customer Service

Why, you may ask, have I written a chapter on customer service? Patients aren't customers are they? Well, the real secret to having a world class Podiatry clinic that provides you with enough profit to live the life that you want while also providing your patients with the best quality medical care is to have good quality customer service.

A customer service that Wows your patients

If you think about the customer service that you receive day to day, as you go about your life, going into shops, cafes and so on we find that in the Western world nowadays Customer service is usually pretty shoddy at best. Therefore, if you can deliver a great customer service, you're already ahead of the game. I strongly recommend, however, that you strive for a wow customer service.

When we are training University, we are primarily being trained to work in the health system and in the health system patients are looked on as patient's only, never customers. Even patients themselves assume themselves to be patients rather than customers when they engage with public health systems and will forgive a poorer quality of customer service

In the private sector, it's a different story altogether. In your patients view, if you're accepting accepting payment from them for your service then they are customers as well as patients and they expect a good quality customer service. It continues to be the case that in the private health sector including Podiatry clinics that customer service is often the last thing that is thought about.

Some podiatrists in private practice believe, without actually realising that they think this way, that the patient they are seeing is the same type of patient that is seen in the free/subsidised public health system. Often these same podiatrists are under the impression that you should never look at the patient as a customer even though the modern fee paying patients believe this to be the case.

I have met some clinicians who have the mindset that to consider providing customer service is somehow not necessary. This is crazy thinking if you are expecting those same patients to pay you their hard earned money for your services.

You need to cherish your patients as both patients and as customers who deserve good customer service in all of their dealings with your clinic. If it wasn't for them deciding to trust you with their health you would not be able to potentially live the lifestyle you desire and do the job you want in an environment that allows you to have personal and financial freedom others don't have.

Think about the last time that you personally got good quality customer service, so good that you had to go home and tell someone about it.

Recently, my wife went to get her haircut. When she went in, she was met by the owner of the salon, who welcomed her by name, asked her how I was getting on with my business even though I've never met him and about our kids all while she sat down having her hair done. She was given a glass of prosecco to drink while reading the latest magazine. All of this made her come home and tell me, who can't tell a fringe cut from a bob cut, all about it. She also told my sister who happened to call that day, strongly recommending that hairdresser to her.

When we get poor customer service we tend to talk about it even more than good customer service don't we. In the past month I went to one of those high street stores that we see everywhere that sell computers. I knew what I wanted and I was happy to spend hundreds of euros. However, I couldn't get anyone to give me the time of day, they were all too busy talking to each other or scrolling to their phones. After 15 minutes I left the shop having spoken to no customer service agent. I instead went online, bought my computer which was delivered the next day. This multinational has since put out a profit warning. No wonder if they can't even get the basics of customer service right. In fact, the customer service was so poor, that here I am talking about it in this book.

The truth is that us humans are not rational. We buy emotionally and we rationalize it later.

You can read more about this in Dan Ariely's book "Predictably Irrational".

When we make any purchasing decision, it's primarily based on emotion in the short term. Why else would people spend more money than need to own a car when a perfectly cheap car can get them can do the job and get them from A to B?

Why do people stay overnight on the street to buy a phone.

It's because the emotion of the object is driving them to make that decision. They'll rationalise it later, they might say I needed that car for safety, or I needed that phone because I just had to download certain podcasts. In most cases, there's usually a cheaper simpler option, but emotional behaviour overrules rational thought when we make any purchasing decisions.

The exact same thing happens when your potential patient decides if they will come to see you and then once you give advice, make a decision on whether or not they will proceed with the treatment you suggest. You need to remember this with regards to all interactions you have with your patient's if you are to get greater buy in from them. I discuss this more in the next chapter.

If you can make sure that the emotional goals of your patients are met and or in a simpler way they left with a good feeling about your clinic, then they will be more likely to come back. They will be more likely to follow through with your plan of care and they will achieve the outcome that they wished when they first contacted you.

Good quality or even exceptional customer service is *the* key to running a profitable clinic.

Obviously, good quality or best practice clinical care is vital, that's a given, but we need to provide more than this in today's competitive market to truly stand out from the crowd. Your patients or customers do not know the difference between one type of treatment you provide and another. All they know is whether they trust you or not to proceed.

Your aim should be to WOW your patients whenever they have any interaction with your clinic, be that in the clinic, on the phone, by email, or with all of your marketing. In my clinic I regularly ask my staff who did you WOW today. My staff understand that every single interaction they have with their patients should deliver exceptional customer service.

Premium customer service allows you to charge a premium price, which is what you need to do to truly have a profitable

Podiatry clinic that is not fully reliant on you. Somebody needs to provide a premium service so that may as well be your clinic.

It's very difficult, if not impossible, to free yourself from your clinic, while still providing the type of profit and lifestyle that you need to earn more and work less if you are the cheapest in town. This is why I have decided to offer a premium customer service type model with a product premium price model to match.

Yes, my clinic is expensive but I make sure we deliver both in terms of customer service and medical outcomes. You should aim to do the same.

There are lots of simple and cost effective ways you can provide exceptional customer service.

Every new patient that comes to my clinic gets a thank you letter personally signed by me which is accompanied by an upsell letter explaining all the other services we do. We also give them two vouchers that they can pass on to family members for a free assessment. *I will talk about this later on in the Internal Marketing chapter.*

When my patients arrive, they arrive into a clinic that has a friendly warm waiting room with soft furnishings and relaxing music. Every single patient that arrives is offered tea and coffee in a china cup, not a chipped mug.

As a side note, we offer Coffee/Tea this for two reasons. The first is that it is good quality customer service and secondly, when that patient accepts the tea or coffee research tells us that due to the theory of reciprocation they are more likely to accept the treatment plan recommended to them and therefore, more likely to achieve their goals that they have. In turn they are more likely to be satisfied with the treatment we provided them with and recommend us to their loved ones.

Not too long ago, I moved my clinic about 15 minutes away on foot from our previous location. One patient had to walk to the clinic and it took her 30 minutes as she got lost. She was late for her appointment, so by the time she was seen it was an hour and a half on since she had begun her journey. She came out of the appointment and asked could she stay for a little longer and have another coffee as the clinic was so pleasant. She told me that she wouldn't mind sitting down and relaxing before she restarted her day as it was such a nice place to hang out. Remember this is the waiting room of medical clinic.

There isn't a day goes by that a patient doesn't ask us what music is playing in the clinic as it's so relaxing and they'd love to have it playing in their home.

The appearance of your clinic is hugely important. You have to remember that your patients don't truly understand the techniques that you're performing. Instead what they judge your clinic on is how the clinic is physically presented.

The furniture, how pleasant your staff are or is the clinic even clean.

Has it been freshly painted?

Have you nice framed pictures on the wall instead of ugly anatomical charts?

Is the carpet they walk on warm and thick?

Is there free parking?

Are you open early and late or even on the weekends?

You need to Disneyfy your clinic. Did you know that Disney paints parts of their parks every two days with a fresh coat of paint to ensure that they deliver an exceptional visual experience to their customers. Now I'm not suggesting that you paint your clinic every two days. What I am suggesting is that you start to sweat the small stuff.

I recently had a staff member go out on his lunch break and change a patient's tire for them. We work longer hours so that our patients don't have to take time off work. We send SMS and email reminders to make sure that they can be assured of not missing that appointment.

In my clinic we enquire of patients after their initial appointment what score they would give us out of 10 and if the score is less than 8 we ring to find out how we could have got a higher score.

We provide gifts at Christmas and Easter to our patients. All the children that come in for the week before Easter receive Easter eggs.

I've heard of a dentist nearby who provides his patients with a warm towel, like you receive in first class on an aeroplane, after they finished treatment with him. It's the small touches that really matter.

We provide a referral reward system. If a patient comes in and says that their next door neighbour had sent them to us then that next door neighbour gets a gift in the post from us in a gold envelope. The gift is a thank you letter signed by me with a Golden Ticket for a free appointment to see us.

This voucher will never go out of date. I have never received any such gift from any other business that I have referred to.

Have you?

You should check in with your patients after they finish up with you. We perform cancellation and DNA follow up phone calls. In my clinic if a patient is unable to make their appointment or did not attend, they will get a call from their clinician. The clinician is trained to ring that patient to see what happened and provide them with all possible assistance over the phone.

We understand life gets in the way of treatment but that does not mean that we can't follow up and give good quality care even if it's over the phone.

When we dispense our orthotics, we dispense them in good quality reusable bags. We add into our bag a little gift like a packet of sweets. Recently we changed the sweets that we put into the bag and one of our staff members went on for 10 minutes to anyone who would listen to her about the sweets that she receives when she gets her contact lenses from an online retailer. She spends €400 a year on contact lenses but she feels she has to talk about the 10 cent bag of sweets as she receives nothing like this from any of this company's other competitors. It makes them more memorable for her, gives greater loyalty and turns her in a spokeswoman for them.

How your staff dress and their are appearance should matter. This will affect your patient or customers perception of your professionalism and likelihood of trusting you with their treatment. White coats are banned in my clinic. We dress in a shirt and tie and the ladies in the clinic dress like a medical consultant would.

All of these small things all add up to a great customer service experience for your patient's. It is this customer service experience and the potential to deliver a Wow experience that will enable you to differentiate your clinic from all of your competitors who, like most businesses, are delivering an average or bland experience.

The secret to having a podiatry clinic that allows you to earn more while working less is delivering a superior customer service to that of your competitors on a consistent and reliable basis and is a sure fire path to boosting your clinics ultimate success.

SECRET NO 4.

Fix Your Leaky Bucket First

In any clinic there is really only 3 ways to increase your turnover and profits

1. Get more new patients

2. Get the patients who have already been to your clinic to come more often

3. Get the patients you have the spend more.

This secret and the next secret, "Internal Marketing Is Simpler By Far" is about getting you to focus on No's 2 & 3 rather than No 1 which is much harder and more expensive for you to implement.

Usually, when I start working with a client in my mentor program, the first thing they want to do is to start external marketing. They want more new patients, as they feel that that is the answer to all of their troubles. That they feel will get them out of the bind they are in whereby they feel they are tied to their business a business that is reliant on the owner completely.

However, this is not a good place to start. Are you aware that is estimated that it costs upwards of 12 times more to get a new patients to come to your business than it is to get a previous patient to come back, or a current patient to complete their current plan of care.

Think of your clinic as a bucket that you pour water(new patients) into. If this bucket is full of holes(such as patients not completing their plan of care) all your effort at getting those new patients will go to waste and you will not make the most of the opportunity provided by your existing patients.

Instead of focusing on those shiny new patients that you hope to attract, focus your attention on the patients you already have.

Sit down and make a list of how you can encourage those patients you already have to spend more in your clinic and come back more often.

- **Is time to raise to raise your prices?**

- **Would some patients benefit from coming back a little sooner?**

- **Can you sell your patients stock items they need anyway such as creams or footwear?**

- **What additional services are you not providing that your existing patients would use.**

A few years after opening my first podiatry clinic I got sick of referring patients on for physio and not getting any notification from the physio's as to what they were doing with my patients. I did my numbers and believed this was a service I my clinic could provide, so I recruited a physiotherapist, opened Keep Active Therapy and increased the size of my business at almost no extra cost.

I had measured how much I was referring out over a 3 month period before I made the decision and knew it would pay for itself. It was profitable very quickly and instead of having 1 business I now had 2 and was providing an extra service to my existing patients at no extra marketing cost.

In my clinics I have introduced a system whereby the clinical staff must walk the patient to the front desk and hand over the patient to the front desk explaining when the patient should come back. This simple measure reduced massively the amount of patients saying "I'll call you when I know my schedule" and not doing so and our rebooking rate shot through the roof and is usually over 80%+.

Another leak to consider is your cancellation policy. Do you even have one, and if you do, are your patients aware of it? When we implemented our policy and made it clear to patients our cancellation rates changed and we noticed rather than cancel fully, patients would rebook for a day later in the week.

So you see,before you go spending money you probably can't spare on Facebook, google ads etc look at your leaky bucket and fix those leaks.

The way I see it, the job of all Podiatrists working in private practice is to help our patients reach their goal. Quite often patients don't know what their goal is to begin with, other than they want to get better. It is my strong belief that if we don't do this, if we don't help them reach that goal, we are failing them and unfortunately this under treatment is endemic in both public and private podiatry clinics.

Under-treatment is in my opinion, equally as unethical as over treatment. Our job is to get that patient to their goal to help them to become the healthiest they can possibly be. In University, we got little or no guidance on how often we should see a patient, how long those appointments should be and how far apart those appointments should have.

What we tend to do when we set up our own clinic is copy what we've seen in other clinics, or the "industry standard". Normally we just copy the clinic we worked in last..... same pricing structure, same number of appointments and so forth.

This "industry standard" tends to consist of one appointment at a time and see how we go. Unfortunately the feedback I've received from patients from the clinics I've worked with are they don't like this model at all. They don't like not knowing what's going on and when the whole process is going to finish.

This model has always irritated me, I couldn't understand how it sort of seemed okay to expect the patient to just wait and see how it went. We expect patients to just put up with it, and just keep paying for appointments, which without giving them any attempt at certainty of when their treatment would end or when it we expect them to reach their goal, if we even know what their goal is.

You wouldn't drop your car in to have it fixed to the local garage because of a noise you heard in the engine and say to the garage owner.. "just see how you go, and I'll pay whatever the bill is at the end". You would expect the garage to carry out an assessment on the engine and give you a call, give you a diagnosis on the issue, give you a full treatment plan and tell you the price *before* they started the work. That would give you the customer enough information to make an educated decision on whether or not you want to proceed with that garage fixing your car.

This seems perfectly rational in most businesses, but for some reason, in health care clinics like podiatry, physiotherapy, and so forth, just doesn't occur. We seem to think that it's perfectly reasonable to let the patient drift along from appointment to appointment, without giving them some sort of guidance on when we expect we should be able to discharge them because they have reached their goal.

Its unsurprising that as a result of this patients tend to either not begin their recommended treatment or begin with drop off quite quickly. Think about those patients who do not follow the treatment plan as you might have designed on day one, perhaps only coming once every two or three appointments, taking longer to get better, and causing frustration for both you and the patient.

Pretty much every coaching client I work with at the start has no idea what percentage of their patients complete their plan of care or reach their goal. Often they're shocked when they check these statistics and when they realise that they don't even find out what is their patient's interpretations of success ie what their goals are.

When I first checked this in my physiotherapy clinic, which I had suspicions was not performing as well as I expected regarding what percent of patients reached their goal, I was very disappointed to find out it was less than 50%. It was 44% in one individual clinicians case.

This issue is endemic in our professions. When staff start to work with me, I make clear to them that their aim should be that 90% of the patients will complete their plan of care, reach the goal that they inform us they wanted to reach on the first appointment, get back active and are fully satisfied with the value of the treatment that they received.

To do this, essentially, you need to do two things. Firstly you need to provide best practice medical care and clinical care. This is a given. If you're not doing this, no matter what you do your business will never succeed. That's not what this book is about.

Secondly, you need buy in from the patient on the need for this plan of care and the need to stick all the way through with the plan to the end. We need great compliance from patients. Any less than this and we will not achieve the patient's goals when they first picked up the phone or contacted you and in my view we have failed that patient.

I want patients in my clinic getting 100% better, not 60%, not 70% better. Too often patients drop off 50% of the way through through a plan of care as they fail to see the value of continuing with the treatment, or justifying spending anymore.They cancel or do not attend.

How frustrating does this make you feel? It drives me nuts.

They do this because they have not bought into the reasoning for continuing all the way to the end. Imagine a patient comes into you. And you tell them that you need to see them 6 times and for argument's sake your charge is €50 per appointment. If you see them any less than 6 times, you know, you won't fix them completely and after 3 appointments, they have spent €150 and they cancel because they cannot see the value in coming back and spending another €150.

6 months down the line because you haven't finished their treatment plan, you haven't fixed them completely, the problem reoccurs. They go to another clinic because they feel when they saw you day one, they wasted their money and they are not likely to keep this thought to themselves.

How is this supposed to help you build your business?

Now you might say that this is the patient's fault. I don't agree with this.... the patient doesn't know what they need. You're the expert and it's your responsibility to make sure that they reach their goals when they come see you.

Now, we are trained in college to believe that good clinical care, the use of science and rational arguments to explain why that clinical care is needed is all you will need to get a patient better.

This is not true, good clinical care is not enough to run a profitable podiatry clinic.

Human beings are not rational. If you've been working with the public for more than six months you'll know this to be true. Simply because you advise a plan of care based on empirical evidence to resolve their issue or it totally rational to come back and see you when you advise does not mean that that patient sitting in front of you will agree and will proceed with that treatment.

We need to accept this and we need to learn the skills to overcome this irrationality. The problem is we have no clue how to speak to patients in a way that helps them overcome their barriers to being compliant. We are not trained in how to consider their fears and most importantly how to sell them on why they need to continue with our plan of care.

Too often I see clinicians declare that they would never sell a treatment plan. They feel that selling is somehow unethical or that it's beneath them. Well guess what?

If you want a successful and profitable podiatry clinic full of satisfied patients that get 100% better, don't cancel and tell all of their friends how good your clinic is, you had better learn how to sell your treatment plans.

I'm assuming that when you gave that patient that appointment it was necessary for them to get better. If they cancel that appointment you felt was appropriate for some reason they will not progress right?

How then can you explain why cancelling that appointment and not following through on the treatment is acceptable to you? I believe that it's not acceptable and you should do all in your power to prevent it because if they cancel it could be argued that you have failed that patient and not delivered on the promise that you could help them get better.

You might say I'm being unfair. Maybe I am, but I'm trying to emphasise how important it is that we get better at explaining to patients and using any and all tools and skills available to us to help us get better compliance from our patients with their treatment plan ensuring they follow their plan of care all the way to the end and hence that we allow them to reach their goals fully.

A mentor of mine once told me that our job is to influence our patient's ethically by helping them to make the correct decision to ensure they live a fully active and healthy life. Any less and we are failing them.

At this point I know some reading this are recoiling at what they believe is the immoral practice of selling a treatment plan. To that I say grow up. As a podiatrist your whole raison d'etre is to get patient's 100% better and that will ONLY happen if they do what you need them to.

So how do you get a patient to commit to a plan of care and to follow all the way through to the end of that plan of care?

Well, what we do is we provide our patient with an action plan or a written report. You'll find a copy of this action plan in my bonus section for buyers of this book at this link www.morepracticeprofits.com/podiatry-business-book-bonus

I want 100% of my patients going home with a written report which details what they have, why they have it and what they need to do to get better. This I believe is what the patient is looking for. All patients in the clinic get this regardless of the condition that they have or the cost of the treatment that they need. Even if a patient does not require any further treatment they still get a report.

To begin with, we firstly find out what the patient's emotional goal is. What we mean by this is what they want to achieve by coming to see us, not just today, but over the course of their treatment. For example, we may have a lady in her 60's who can no longer go for a walk with her husband in the evenings or struggling to keep up with their grand-kids. This is her emotional goal.

Getting rid of the pain in her foot is not her emotional goal, that is her more rational goal.

Why do we do act like this?

We do so because when people buy something or make a decision on buying something, they make an emotional decision first. They then rationalise it later.

We then go on to explain to them what they have and why they have it. We use our clinical training but we also make sure to use plain language to do so. Patients don't need to hear too many scientific terms as they will tend to turn off or disengage which is not going to lead to good compliance is it? Following this, we detail to them the treatment plan needed.

Too often the patient goes home and has no idea what happened in the appointment. A conversation at home after the appointment might go something like this;

Spouse: Well, what do you have?

Patient: Well, I have some sort of problem with my foot. I'm not too sure what it is exactly, it's a big and complicated name.

Spouse: Okay, so what you need to do to get it better?

Patient: I'm not sure but I just have to go back the next day.

Spouse: Did he tell you how long it would take to get you better?

Patient: Sort of.

Spouse: Did he tell you what the total cost of sorting it is?

Patient: No.

Spouse: That doesn't sound like a great clinic to me. Why don't try that new clinic in town, they seem to be cheap at least?

Patient: I'll go back and see how I get on. I'll give him one or two appointments and if I'm not sorted I'll try that other clinic.

This type of thing drives me totally bananas.Every patient should be clear on what they have, why they have it and what it takes to fix them.

Our job during an initial appointment is to give the patient all the information that they need to overcome any objections or doubts that they may have had on why not to go ahead with treatment and not to follow the care plan all the way to the end. Anything less than this, we are not going to help that patient get full resolution of their symptoms and therefore I believe we have let them down.

The key to all of this is your patients emotional goal.

Your patient doesn't care about their range of motion of their ankle or whether they are pronating or supinating or if their subtalar joint is medially deviated. Really all they care about is getting back for a walk with their husband, or being able to keep up with their grandchild or completing that 5km run.

That 5km run or walking with their husband is their emotional goal and what they consciously or subconsciously focus on to make a buying decision. You need to use this in your conversation with them to ensure that they embark on and then fully complete their plan of care.

The way I see it is *your* responsibility to use this knowledge to help your patient reach their goals and live a healthier life. You should continue to discuss their emotional goals throughout their initial appointment as you attempting to persuade your patient on the most appropriate plan of care.

Think about it.... When you last bought that handbag or smartphone or, if you are like me, equipment for your favourite sport. You in all likelihood didn't really need it but you emotionally wanted it and you convinced yourself after you had made the purchase that it was the right decision.

We make our buying decisions emotionally and rationalise it afterwards and this is also unfortunately true when it comes to the health care purchases your patient's make in your clinic. I know you probably wish that this was not how people act when it comes to the choices they will make in relation to your advice. However it is this aspect of human behaviour that makes people sleep out all night to get the new smartphone or for the New Years sales.

The great thing about the science of human behaviour is you can study the research and use it in your daily interaction with people and influence them to make better decisions that will lead to better health care at your clinic.

Your patients at this point will have three main questions.

No1; What is happening to cause my issue?

No2; What's it going to take to get it sorted and allow them to reach their goal?

No3; What's the total cost going to be?

Most clinicians are pretty good at No 1 and No 2 but we tend to avoid No 3 like the plague? We find it very uncomfortable to talk about money.

It's drummed into us University, that charging for Medicare is not a good thing to aspire to but it's pretty hard to run a private practice if we're not going to charge our patients. In *Secret 5 You Need A Robust Price Strategy*,I discuss in more detail forming a pricing structure.

Our discomfort with talking about money is often the reason why we take the easy option and go for that one appointment at a time technique, which leads to patients tending to cancel after a few appointments as they have no idea when this is going to stop.

If you can get your patients to commit to a plan of care to begin with, to see it through to the end, you will deliver greater results, patient satisfaction, encourage greater word of mouth referrals, substantially improve your clinics cash flow and profit in an ethical way.

You owe it to your patients to get better at selling.

If this makes you uncomfortable, then think of it as getting better at convincing your patients what's needed to get them to get 100% better.

This approach will help you to eliminate or significantly reduce drop offs, cancellations and DNA's from patients. There's nothing I hate more than to see a patient that is cancelled or not turn up for an appointment when I know I could have done more gotten further along. I never blame the patient, I always blame myself that I did not convince them well enough that they needed to turn up for that appointment.

Before spending your hard earned money on marketing to get new patient's first get the patients you already have to come more often by simply sticking to their treatment plan.

Make the most of the patient's you already have by providing them with better quality of care, exceptional customer service and getting them 100% not 75% better.

The secret to running a profitable Podiatry clinic is to get better at influencing patient's to make the right decisions.

SECRET NO 5.

You Need A Robust Price Strategy

This is a scary subject for most health professionals and one we avoid if we can. It makes us feel very uncomfortable to think about the prices we charge. How do we decide how to charge a patient?

We don't want to come across as money grabbing, but at the same time, we need to charge our patients something. The prices we charge is a subject the majority Podiatry clinic owners spend the least amount of time they can on which is a bit odd really for a business.

To be clear at the start, this Secret No 5 is about working out what's the correct strategy for you to decide your pricing model. This is not about trying to gouge money out of patients or charging more than you feel comfortable with. However it is the truth that price does drive your clinics profit and profit in turn determines how successful your clinic will be and the level of financial and personal freedom you achieve.

How great would it feel to have a clinic that delivers exceptional medical care, brilliant customer service and is full of fulfilled staff giving their best to their patient's whilst giving you the lifestyle you wanted when you first started your clinic?

How great would it be to have a clinic that gives you the freedom to choose how much work you do that week?

Wouldn't you like to have podiatry clinic that is a real business, not just a job, that you can sell on at a great price when you are ready. A healthy profit will give you just that and that healthy profit only comes from the right pricing structure.

The appropriate profit *(I go into detail on how to work out your P&L in Secret No 6)* does one main thing. It gives you and your business choices. Choices on investing in your people, investing in training, investing in marketing, newer & better equipment, more of the services your patients want and are happy to pay for.

A healthy profit gives you choices on the type of lifestyle and work life balance you the clinic owner want.

But Lorcan, *"My patients are different. They won't pay higher prices",* I hear you say.

Yes, there are some patients no matter what will complain about the price that you charge. You know the type of patient I'm talking about. Even if it was free, this type of patient would still complain. This type of patient will choose their healthcare solely based on the ability to avoid any financial cost to them regardless of the quality of the care that's provided.

However, just as equally for every one of those type of patient's there is another one who is happy to pay more for your service. The type of patient who turns up on time, always pays their bill, is compliant and a pleasure to work with. I know which type I would like to work with.

You have a choice to make as the owner of your own clinic/business. Do you continue worrying about not being seen to charge too much and suffer the consequences of not making enough profit? Or do you decide that you don't want to take all the hassle of your clinic, sleepless nights, pressure of wages, rent, consumables and begin to charge the correct price that provides you with the profit you need.

If you want to have a business that does not provide you with sufficient income, why not just go and get a job in the public health service and save yourself the stress. However, if you want to be in business, then act like you are running a business, not a charity and set your prices appropriately for that business.

What use are you to your patients if you don't bring in enough income to keep the doors open? You won't help anyone that way. As clinicians we worry more about the price we charge for our services than most of our patients do.

How do most clinic owners set their prices?

I bet when you set your prices on the first day when you opened your clinic you probably did one of the following;

Number 1: You looked at what other clinics locally charged and decided to charge the average.

Number 2: You asked friends,family or prospective clients what they were willing to pay.

Number 3: You figured out your costs and you added just a little bit for profit.

Number 4: You just guessed what might work.

Most clients that I work with have used option 1. They don't want to be the most expensive, they don't want to be the cheapest. They don't know what to do so they go for the middle price point in their area.

Why do we do this sort of stuff as health practitioners? The truth is, we are afraid. Fear drives most decisions when it comes to setting price. We're afraid that we will be seen as being greedy or that we are only concerned with making money by our peers. Usually we are more worried about what our peers might think rather than joe public.

I understand this. This comes from my from our training. I did the very same thing and it almost cost me my business. What use would I have been to my patients if I had gone bust because I wasn't able to charge the right price? Since I realised that my prices where just too low to survive never mind thrive and that price is elastic I have increased my prices every year.

I find that the higher my prices are the less that I get complaints from patients about price. This is due to 2 main reasons. To begin with my pricing strategy attracts the type of patient's who are happy to pay, appreciate the work we do and are more compliant and because secondly I make sure that my clinic delivers on the price that we charge.

So how should you set your prices. Price of any service or item is far more elastic than we realise. People are happy to pay a premium price for something if they are satisfied of the perceived value. Take note I say perceived value. This is subjective. If they feel the outcome eg; *"getting back walking"* is worth the cost, not just a financial cost, they will be happy to pay us.

Remember, it is an emotional not a rational decision. Why else do people buy that expensive handbag or that car that's too big for their driveway? I recently heard that 50% of Americans never have $1,000 saved at any time in their life. Yet, the significant portion(81%) of the very same people have a smartphone work over $1,000.

Rationally this makes no sense. Surely they could have bought a much cheaper phone that pretty much does the same thing?

Why does this happen?

It happens because we are not rational beings. We make our buying decisions mostly based on emotion. The exact same thing is true when it comes to making decisions in healthcare.

I have 4 children and all of them were born in the local maternity hospital on the public system. All of the healthcare both my wife and kids got was 100% free and I must say exceptional. The funny thing is you can pay to have almost the exact same care in the exact same hospital by the exact same midwives nurses etc. The cost is about €5,000 per child and the place is full of couples happy to pay this fee as they perceive it must be better care because its more expensive.

Now I think this is a total waste of money, €20,000 if my wife and I did this. However I understand that everyone including me has things they absolutely will not spend a higher price for and certain services they will. The mistake almost all small business owners including podiatry clinic owners make is they project their own opinion of what they would be willing to pay for their services on to their customers.

Just because you would not spend this money on a service does not mean others wouldn't be more than happy to do so. When setting your prices do not assume that your or you peers opinion on a maximum price you can charge is the absolute truth. You and other medics are often coming from a place where the ethos was that charging for medical care is somehow unethical. Usually these views are provided by those who have a stable wage packet at the end of every month and have never taken the risk of opening their own clinic and living off the results.

The first thing I do with my mentoring clients is I get them to put their price up straight away. Usually this suggestion is a shock to them and I met with a lot of resistance. Often this debate can last for weeks or even months and eventually, the prices go up by a little bit (less than I advised). On the next call, I ask my mentoring clients have they had any complaints and 99% of the time there was absolutely no issue with the price rise from patient's and the clinic owners regrets not doing so a lot sooner.

In most cases it dawns on the clinic owner that they have just had their minds opened to the reality of the elasticity of price and that perhaps they've been undervaluing their services for longer than they care to admit.

They admit that patients are quite happy to pay a higher price if they perceived value to be worth that price.

Our next step after this is to work out how much profit they need. We determine what their goals are in their life, over the next 12 months, three years, five years and so on.

We then figure the cost of achieving their goals.

The business's job is then to ensure that these personal and professional aims are fulfilled and how much profit is needed to make sure that this occurs.

My belief is that we should work to live not live to work.

Now don't get me wrong I work very hard my wife says too hard, but I want to be rewarded for that. For too long, I worked very hard with little or no real financial reward. I never felt it was never worth it. I was burnt out, stressed all of the time and could see little point in continuing to run the businesses as I did.

In my own clinic working backwards, like I do with my coaching clients, I decide what profit I want over the next 12 months and therefore each month and where we need to set our prices to achieve this accordingly.

Obviously, you need to be realistic. You can't go from a business that makes a profit of €10,000 per year to a business that makes a profit of €1,000,000 a year overnight. You should start to test the possibilities of price elasticity in your clinic. In regard to most of the services you provide, you will find that your patient's price elasticity stretches much further than you expected it to.

Remember it's not you or your opinion regarding price that you are trying to attract as a patient. Personally I would prefer to work all day with patient's who were happy to pay me well for a great quality service than those who simply wanted the cheapest price.

The secret of a profitable podiatry business is that you too can choose what kind of patient's you want to work with using a great pricing strategy.

SECRET NO 6.

You Have Got To Know Your Numbers.

As with any business, knowing your numbers is vital. If you don't know what profits you've made or what your turnover was and so forth, how can you make any educated decisions about the financial health or otherwise of your business.

Just like when a patient comes to us with a musculoskeletal injury, we'd like to check the flexibility, the range of motion and so on. We do this because we can compare it to others and we can make comparisons going forward and determine if things are moving in the right direction.

When I ask any new clients of mine in my coaching business what their profit was as a percentage of their turnover in the last quarter there's often silence on the phone. God forbid if I asked them what the patient acquisition costs are or a simple but vital statistic such as what's their lifetime customer spend? I would predict that the number of clinic owners that know these answers is very very small.

I was the same once upon a time. I had absolutely no clue of my numbers. In Ireland, where I live, when you're self employed you pay your tax in early November, for the year before. I used to meet my accountant in mid October where we'd spend an hour chatting mostly about sport the weather and his passion..... art. Then maybe the last 10 minutes we'd spend talking about his bill for the work he had done for me. Finally we turn our attention to whole reason for the meeting .... the tax bill that I had incurred on the profit made in the previous calendar year.

I would walk out with my head swimming, not knowing why I had such a large tax bill considering I had no money left at the end of any month. I would go home and panic for approximately two weeks while I tried to figure out why my tax was so high and how I was going to come up with the money to pay for it.

I managed to kick this "Tax Bill" can down the road for a number of years but eventually, the result was that I ended up with a tax bill greater than the profit from the year before. With no ability to pay it the banks would not touch me as they could see I had did not have a handle on my business. I had swiftly to move to a new accountant who had to negotiate with the revenue and ultimately the city Sheriff a payment plan so I would be able to keep my doors open.

It was the most stressful situation I had ever found myself in in my whole life and I promised myself I would never let that happen again. The change I decided I would make was I would always know my numbers in detail from now on. I now know my numbers in real time. Not only that but I'm able to tell what profit we made the week before or my cash flow, my turnover, and so forth.

What happens if you don't know your numbers?

Imagine flying a plane with no dashboard in the cockpit giving you information about the planes performance. It's fine as long as you stay up and running but if you run out of petrol, try to land or climb higher you're in danger of crashing as you have no idea what's happening outside your cockpit.

The same happens with your business. If you try to scale up or even maintain the status quo of your business without knowing your figures you are at severe danger of crashing your business and potentially at some point running into the reality of lack of cash flow. I hope you can see it's imperative that you know your numbers before you proceed any further with marketing, etc.

How to Choose your accountant.

If you have an accountant relationship like I had initially then it's time you've considered moving elsewhere. When beginning to decide what accountant to choose you need to ask around all the successful businesses or clinic owners you know for some recommendations. Then interview all of your potential accountants. Take your time and work out what you want to know before you meet them.

Don't be afraid to ask lots of questions, its should be you interviewing them for the job, not the other way around. Your accountant should ideally be able to give you advice on how to maximise your tax efficiency. Whoever you choose should be able to help you plan in advance to avoid any nasty surprises when it comes to your tax.

They should be able to mentor you on how to manage your cash flow, your profit and loss, how to read a balance sheet and so on. Ask them will they the right person to help you with building the wealth that comes with scaling your business.

In essence your accountants job is to help you maximise your financial health.

My accountant does all of this for me. We have regular financial health checks, quarterly meetings which include a balance sheet and his profit & loss statements. We continually have tax planning with updates on this weekly. We also discuss long term wealth planning with a focus on my financial goals.

If you have an accountant that doesn't do any of these things, that simply gives you his bill and tells you your tax bill with minimal advice then you need to consider a change as soon as possible.

Tax planning

In conjunction with your accountant, you should plan for any tax bills due well in advance. The best method is to have your accountant/bookkeeper advise you with lots of notice the tax you should expect to pay. This will allow you to put this money aside. I recommend that you put money aside into a bank account that is hard to reach. This will mean it will be harder for you to dip into this when you when you feel the need, such as in a cash flow pinch. If you can predict your tax bill you can plan for it.

One of the biggest mistakes I have ever made as I explained was in relation to tax. What got me into all my trouble was I paid my staff a percentage of their turnover like most of my peers. As I couldn't predict their turnover every week, it was very difficult to predict their tax and my employers tax liabilities that would fall due.

While my old accountant did not help much with this I have to admit I had my head in the sand.

Key Performance Indicators.

Key performance indicators are the numbers that tell you how your businesses performing from day to day week to week. They are like the dials in the cockpit of your plane.

The more dials you have and the more current and accurate they are the better for your business. Your KPI's will allow you to compare your profitability, turnover, utilisation rate (how full you are), wages as a percent of turnover and so on and therefore take action when they are not meeting your expectations.

An example of this in a clinical setting would be doing a lunge test/ankle dorsiflexion measurement on every patient that comes in with a musculoskeletal issue that you feel is related to a lack of ankle movement. If appropriate you would set in place a treatment plan to improve the patient's ankle range of motion and retest at regular intervals so you can see an improvement. This would be an example of a key performance indicators with regards to this patient.

Ideally you should be able to know in real time what our key performance indicators are. Most CRM software systems used in modern podiatry clinics will give you some KPI's. I have yet to find one that of these CRM systems that gives enough of the KPI's you really really need and you will have to to develop procedures to deliver KPI's your clinic will require.

Some of the key performance indicators that I recommend you know are ;

1. Number of new patients weekly and monthly.

2. Number of consults weekly

3. Monthly percentage of new patients who book a second follow up appointment

4. Utilisation rate or the percentage of your clinicians time that is spent face to face with patients. This is important as it lets you know when you were running an efficient clinic and are ready to scale up or take on new staff.

5. The average number of appointments advised in advance by your by your staff. This should be broken down by appointment type.

6. The average number of those appointments advised that were booked by those patients. Again this should be broken down by appointment type.

7. Turnover per staff member, daily, weekly, monthly and yearly. This should be compared from staff member to staff member.

8. Average lifetime value of your patients per initial appointment type. This lets you know how much you should expect to turnover for each type of appointment.

9. Patient acquisition costs per marketing channel and per appointment type. In a podiatry clinic, if you find that it costs you €50 to acquire a chiropody patient, and that patients only spends €50 that's not going to grow your business by much. That marketing channel needs to improve by becoming cheaper at acquiring that type of patient.

10. Break even point per day, per week, per month and per year. If you don't know what it costs to break even every day, you have no way of knowing if your business is in the red or black on a daily basis.

11. Percentage of the staff wage versus turnover for every staff member. This will help you see who is performing and what staff are being carried by the others.

12. Number of leads per marketing funnel & percentage of conversion of those leads & turnover per lead/conversion.

13. Number of patient's that cancel with no follow up made & DNA appointments.

All of these KPIs reduce or remove the subjectivity of how your business is performing, and instead gives you objectivity. This means that when you find something that's not as it should be, you are able to act quickly and have the information for your staff at hand to show that this is entirely accurate. This is important to get buy in from your stuff. If they can see that it's not your opinion but rather the figures/facts they are more likely to help you address and work on the issue.

Profit and Loss.

Profit and Loss is a very important way of knowing how healthy your business is performing. This is different from an accountants balance sheet or his P&L. Your accountant should be doing a P&L but you should also do your own version, as your accountants is primarily focused on your tax bill and minimising it.

I would advise doing your own P&L monthly and I insist that all of my coaching clients do so. How I have them do it is as follow;

1. They record their turnover for each clinic location. If they have 2 types of clinic in the one location this is separated. An example of this might be a podiatry clinic that also runs a physiotherapy clinic out of the same location.

2. Next, they record the wage cost per department in that clinic. They then record the owner wage or what it would cost to replace the owners clinical hours if they were to employ another clinician to replace the owners clinical work. This is often quite revealing as it in almost all cases shows that the owner can reduce their clinical hours significantly at a much lower cost than most owners realised before they did the numbers.This is important information to allow you the owner to begin the process of replacing yourself.

3. The next step is they should record their costs and this should be as detailed as possible. For example, marketing shouldn't be broken down into each type of marketing. With regards to cost, you should avoid putting anything into this that is not strictly needed for running the clinic.

Large purchases or payments, such as a large piece of equipment should be spread over at least 12 calendar months. If you were to put these large costs into one single month it will skew your figures markedly.

4. You should then be able to calculate your profit as a percentage of your turnover, your wages as a percentage of your turnover, your costs as a percentage of your turnover and your owners wage as a percentage of turnover.

Doing your P&L like this will allow you see where your costs are higher or lower than the ideal and act accordingly. They will also help you to replace yourself over time by developing and leveraging systems (see Secret 12). Profit and Loss gives you information the other accounting type reports simply do not.

At one point I had a coaching client who had multiple clinics and spent most of her time and effort on one in particular. Once she had done her first profit loss, she realized that this clinic, which was taking approximately 65% of her time while only providing her with 37% of her profits. This allowed us to alter her priorities when it came to her clinics and boost her profits without the need for further external marketing spend.

Long term financial planning.

While this book is not designed to give long term financial advice I feel that too many podiatry clinic owners are living for today only. Often they feel if they just keep working like mad eventually it will all pay off financially when it comes time to retire or sell the business. In an effort to help the business they put all the spare cash straight back into the business and in essence put all of their eggs in one basket.

I would suggest you get your hands on the book *"Profit First"* by Mike Michalowicz. In the book the author makes the premise that business owners move a small percentage of the business's turnover into a separate, difficult to access, account before paying any bills. The idea is take the profit first. He suggests starting at 1% as this will allow you to run your business with the remaining 99% thereby avoiding a sudden cash flow shock and over time building up the profit first percentage. This money is then used to invest in other assets both for now and the future ensuring your business runs more efficiently and you are spreading your risk into other investment opportunities.

I hope you can see from this chapter that if you are like I was at one time, only vaguely knowing your numbers or getting your figures from your accountant once a year then you are not really in charge of the levers affecting your business and will be unable to make educated and effective choices to improve your business financial health. If this sounds like you then start by meeting your accountant a little more often, make a plan and begin to measure more things, adding one KPI at a time.

Leasing & Getting Your Rent Right

Negotiating a lease is an art in itself. You almost need to be a poker player, something I am not good at. I strongly advise getting legal advice. When negotiating any lease there should be a balance between security and flexibility.

Security of lease.

You need enough security to make sure that you are not thrown out at short notice as has happened to clients of mine in the past and we've had to scramble to save their business.

Flexibility of lease.

Should you find that you scaled you clinic at such a rapid pace that is impossible to expand in your current premises you will require flexibility in your lease such as option to terminate. An example is a 10 year lease with a 2 and 7 year break clause and a 5 year rent review.

If you can, you should do your very best to avoid a sublease. In a situation like this, if your landlord has not paid the rent to his landlord, whether you pay him or not, it will be you and your business that will be at risk.

As a ballpark, it's recommended that your rent is no more than 10% of your turnover but really you should be aiming for less in a healthcare business. If your marketing is good enough, people will travel to you and you don't necessarily have to have a prime location, especially in the early stages of scaling up when you're trying to protect your cash flow.

I moved my clinic from the city centre to a quiet suburb 3 km away. While we may have had some reservations before moving, making sure all of my current and patient's were aware well in advance of the move and because we had good quality marketing our turnover instead of having any drop increased by 65% in the year following the move.

There's a lot to be said to be able to buy your premises in time. However do not so so if it places undue strain on your cash flow and profitability.

So you see if you don't know your numbers in as close to real time as possible to really cannot make any educated decisions for the good of your business.

The secret to running a profitable podiatry clinic, earning more and working less is knowing your numbers.

SECRET NO 7.

Why Almost All Podiatry Clinics Are Wasting Their Money On Marketing.

So what is marketing anyway? What does marketing mean to you?

Have you ever thought about it? I suspect you haven't put a whole lot of effort into thinking about your marketing or your marketing plan. It's not something we podiatrists have any experience in or had any training for when we come out of college.

The Oxford English Dictionary tells us that *"marketing is the activity of presenting advertising and selling a company's product or services in the best possible way".*

Pause here and read that again.

It says that it is an activity whereby we try to sell our service, ie podiatry in the best possible way. Now you might argue that the best possible way is highly subjective, isn't it?

Well, I don't feel that it should be. I strongly believe that marketing's purpose is to is to fill you and your clinicians diary with the type of patients that you like to treat and are a profitable type of patient to see.

Your marketing should be held accountable. Holding your marketing accountable should mean that your marketing helps you reach the goals that you have set for you and your clinic in as financially efficient a way as is possible.

Let's be honest, when most podiatry clinic owners think of marketing, they think advertising with Google or placing an ad in the paper. You might think that getting likes on Facebook is really what marketing is all about and the answer to all of your clinics problems.

I have met lots of clinic owners who think that it is unethical to market their services for some reason. My little girl has speech and language issues. Once after her speech and language therapy session the owner of the clinic got talking to me. I started to explain to her the kind of marketing that we were doing in our clinic and how much success we were having from it. She made a face and suggested that she couldn't possibly continence doing marketing as she believed it was unethical to do so in healthcare.

My argument was that it was her duty to explain to the public why they needed to come and see her. It was her duty to tell patients like my daughter how her clinic could help her live a better life. I felt it was incumbent upon her and other clinics like hers to make sure that patients like my daughter, who are in need of the best possible medical assistance, are given all of the possible information and assistance that they could get. This should include a commitment from the clinic owner that they will use marketing to explain to prospective patients that their clinic is the right place to get the appropriate help to reach their goals. Anything less than that, in my opinion, is what is unethical.

What's the alternative? Do not inform the public of the services your clinic provides that will improve their quality of life and possibly they have inferior or inappropriate care elsewhere. We have all had patient's come into us whom we knew if we had seen them before they visited another clinic, could have avoided inferior medical care.

I once was attended a weekend CPD course and sat down for lunch with three or four physiotherapists. Two of them said that they had no need for a website as they got all of their work from "word of mouth" and dismissed out of hand the idea that any "good clinic" should ever need one.

This is ridiculous.

In my opinion, we have a responsibility as clinicians to inform our patients of what we do and how we are the right clinic to help them for the particular issues that we are trained to address. We have a responsibility to help build the podiatry profession. Too often I hear clinicians and clinic owners giving out about their professional bodies and how it's their responsibility alone to build the professions in the eyes of the public.

Rubbish I say.

All of us clinic owners have a special responsibility to build our clinics so that they provide for all of its stakeholders. That it provides for its patients, so that they get the best policy quality care. For our staff to ensure that they have good job security and develop a good culture within the clinic itself. For our clinicians so that we can have the turnover to invest in CPD to ensure that they develop to be the best that they can be.

You the clinic owner has a responsibility to yourself to ensure that you receive the financial rewards that you deserve for putting up with all of the stress and hassles that is involved in running and building a successful podiatry clinic. A properly executed marketing plan will allow you to achieve just this.

Clinic owners including myself are in a relatively privileged position as we have the resources and ability at our fingertips to educate and inform the public using marketing. This is normally not possible if you are an employee or work in the health services.

When first I begin discussing marketing with my coaching clients in More Practice Profits I explain to them that marketing is every single interaction that they have with their patients throughout the life's patients life cycle. You should think of marketing as including how you and your staff are dressed, how you greet your patients on the phone and in person.

Marketing is your stationery and your reports to other medics, your business cards, your clinics decor and even its smell or ambience. It's your advertising on Google, Facebook, Instagram, in the newspaper, your website's appearance and its usefulness for the patient. Your marketing is your follow up system.

Think of your marketing as absolutely every single thing that your patient sees, hears, smells and experiences throughout that patients interaction with you and your clinic. This is a different approach to how most clinic consider marketing, how your competitors consider marketing.

So how do most Podiatry clinics market? Well, they think marketing is just advertising. So they put up a website with little to no thought about what it should be doing for business. Most of them tend to look at other Podiatry Clinic websites and copy them, usually the clinic that they aspire to most. They might get a graphic designer, who in reality has no clue about the psychology of decision making online, to build them a website. Most graphic designers like to have a pretty but ineffective website and suggest a similarly pretty but ineffective website design to the Podiatry clinic owner.

These websites are usually packed with lots of nice pictures of feet and so on thinking that this is what will attract the patient.

This Podiatry Clinic owner might open a Facebook page and believe that if they're getting lots of "likes" or "shares" it will be the answer to all of their financial worries. You can't take a Facebook like to the bank. They do the odd blog, which is written in very technical language because that is how they have been taught to write when they come out of University. They buy whatever advertising they are offered by the marketing salesman that contacts them. They might be paying someone to do a bit of SEO, whatever that means but usually they're not too sure if it is bringing in any new patients.

The plain truth is that most podiatric clinic owners have no clue what they are doing. They have no real idea what profit their marketing is making for them or if it's even breaking even at all. These Podiatry clinic owners have no plan and have no idea of how to develop a marketing plan.

These are the kind of Podiatry clinic owners who say, *"marketing hasn't worked for me, I tried Google ads and it doesn't work"* or worst of all, *"My marketing is word of mouth"*. This means they don't know what to do so they dismiss the whole concept.

Some of you reading this may say, *"Well, actually Lorcan, I do have a marketing plan".* But in all likelihood, you are still making the same basic errors. I know this because most small businesses are making the exact same errors. If you look online or you look in your local newspaper, and you will see they're all making the same mistakes. I too made all of these same mistakes for years and wasted more money than I care to admit.

Pause for a moment and imagine the number of people in your local town that have sore feet, (eg; plantar fasciitis) that you know you can help if they just came to your clinic and not your competitors. We believe as clinic owners and as medics that they are all ready to buy now and pick up the phone and come and see us. Surely all you need to do is show them that your clinic "cares" or has better "qualifications" or is "registered" and those patients will automatically pick to come and see you. Well, they don't do they?

These people are just not ready to buy now. Various research suggests that between 3% and 7% of people are ready to buy now when they are looking for a product or service. This percentage of your potential patients with plantar fasciitis are actively searching for someone to solve their heel pain right now. These are the type of people that are calling your clinic on the phone and asking you for an appointment.

The mistake that most clinic owners are making is that they are all chasing only these patients that are ready to buy now.

They're spending all of their marketing budget on this small percentage of the population who are ready to make a decision on who they want to help them with their foot pain today.

They are totally ignoring the other 93 to 97% of people who also have a problem, but are not ready to make a decision on whether to trust someone at all or even where to go to have that help. Almost all Podiatry clinics marketing consists of BOOK NOW or CALL NOW for an appointment.

These clinics fail to realise that most people are simply not ready to book now. These patients are just too sceptical or worried about making a decision and telling them to BOOK NOW, or to look at how much more we care, or how well qualified we are, is never going to overcome their scepticism.

It is inbuilt into humans that making decision comes with risks, so the safest thing to do to avoid this risk is to make no decision or put simply avoiding trusting any clinic by booking that appointment. These potential patients are looking on websites of clinics like yours and the finding they are all the same, that they are full of medical jargon. These websites don't speak to them, or to their worries with regards to who to trust.

As I mentioned these websites are all about the clinic and all about the medical conditions they treat, how great they are, how many courses they've done, their qualifications and the technology that they have in the clinic. I'm sorry to burst your bubble, but these websites are practically useless. The truth is that patients don't really care what qualification you have, how long you've been in college or what letters are after your name.

The only thing these potential patients care about is:

- Can you tell me what I have?

- Can you help me get back to what it's stopping me doing?

- Can you tell me how long it's going to take?

- How can I trust you?

One mentor of mine said to me, patients don't care what you know until they know that you care. However, we don't build our websites with this in mind. We tend to develop our marketing including our website thinking that the best way to convince people to choose us is to explain what we know rather than how we can help that person reach their goal.

Without realising it we make the marketing all about us and not about the patient, their fears, their barriers to making a decision and the factors *they* consider when choosing one clinic over another.

People buy from someone they know, like and they trust. What I help members of my coaching program realise, is they need to allow that sceptical patient ,that 90%+, slowly build a relationship with them so that they can grow to know, like and trust their clinic. I also train them that they need to do so at a pace that the potential patient is comfortable with.

By doing this they gradually have overcome these potential patients understandable scepticism.

Think about patients like this who have come to you in the past. You've explained to them what they have and for some reason they don't go ahead with the treatment even though you were convinced of your diagnosis and confident of a positive outcome from the treatment plan you outlined.

How often has this sort of thing happened to you with patient's you were sure you had made a connection with?

For years I used to find this so frustrating and could never understand how patients were being so irrational. For example, I had a lady, let's call her Maureen, who came to see me a number of years ago. She'd had an issue with her left foot and I explained to her what is was, the reasons for its occurrence and what the treatment plan should be. I advised her that she would need orthotics as part of her plan of care and was very confident of resolving her issue. Maureen laughed, opened up her handbag and took out a Ziploc bag which contained 6 different pairs of orthotics she'd received from 5 different clinics.

How could Maureen be anything but sceptical? Most potential patients like Maureen don't even pick up the phone to clinics like ours, because they've already been to similar clinics and had really poor experiences. Now you might argue that your clinic is different and I'm sure it is, but to all of the Maureen's out there they all look the same because they are all saying the exact same sort of thing. They are all using the same ineffective marketing which does nothing to convince Maureen that your clinic is different from all the other vanilla flavoured clinics.

The key to overcoming scepticism for patients like Maureen is building a relationship with her so that she gets to know, like and trust you and choose your clinic when she's ready to make a decision.

The secret is to combine Information Marketing and Direct Response marketing.

At some point, these sceptical potential patient's are going to have to make a decision about getting help and it might as well be with your clinic they choose because you are the best place to help them. Aren't you?

Information Marketing

Information marketing is marketing whereby you provide information to the potential client/patient up front at little or no cost to them so that you get the chance to start to build a relationship with them directly.

Direct Response

Direct response marketing is marketing where your marketing results in the potential patient responding to the advertisement and then being responded to by the clinic. This can be partially or fully automated.

Let me give you an example of how this process works in my clinic and how I help clients of my coaching programme implement a similar automated system.

Joe Bloggs sits at home on a Saturday night after another week of having a sore foot. His next door neighbour told him that he probably has plantar fasciitis because his sister had the same thing and it was almost impossible to get rid of and make sure to watch out as she ended up shelling out a lot of money in a few places in town that all talk the same fancy talk and never got her sorted. In the end her GP gave her a few injections which helped but she had to give up running for 18 months!

Joe takes out his smartphone and does a google search for Plantar Fasciitis. My ad appears at the top of Google Ads where it talks about Plantar Fasciitis and the area Joe lives in.

Joe clicks on the ad and it brings him to a landing page I have designed that is ONLY about Plantar Fasciitis. The landing page is not all about my clinic and how much we care more or how well we are qualified. On the landing page Joe is given a number of options. He can download for free a report that I have written on some tips that he can use at home to begin to ease his plantar fascia pain immediately.

He can also request a free phone call from one of my clinical team who will discuss his issue and see if we are the right clinic for him. Thirdly, he can request a free 20 minute consultation with one of my podiatry team to again discuss his issue, answer all of his questions and help Joe to overcome any reservations or barriers he may have to beginning any treatment.

I don't ask Joe to pay for anything. Everything is free up front. The barrier to starting his relationship with my clinic is very low.

Go to the bonus section for a free copy of my lead magnet. https://www.morepracticeprofits.com/podiatry-business-book-bonus

Most of the patient's who go through this process will download the free report. In exchange they provide us with their email, their name and their phone number and they are followed up within 24 hours by my administration team, who want to double check to make sure that they got the report and that the report was appropriate for their condition.

They will then initiate a conversation with Joe to see what's been happening and how can we help and Joe will then be offered further help upfront at little or no cost. Often Joe will be invited in for a Free Foot Assessment and from there on we gradually help to break down Joe's scepticism and lay out in front of him a treatment plan that will allow him to reach his goals and rid him of his plantar fasciitis.

Yes, this takes approach of giving information in advance of any payment in exchange for the opportunity to build trust and develop a relationship, is a bit of work and takes time no matter what medium you use. Nowadays a lot of this can be automated and the results are fantastic.

The difference between this and what most clinics are doing is that they will expect Joe to book an appointment straight away and pay for the information he needs to make a decision.

• Joe's not ready for that.

• Joe doesn't know what he has.

• He doesn't know if you're the right clinic.

- He simply doesn't trust you yet.

You're asking him to make too big of a decision, too big of a commitment, so his decision is to make no decision and no commitment as its the safer option.

Instead you should offer Joe a very risk free or minimal risk choice and once he's done that, steadily ... step by step, build a relationship and overcome his barriers to beginning treatment.

As podiatrists we are experts in our field and we have mountains of information between our ears. The mistake that we all make is to expect all patients to simply pick up the phone and arrange to pay for that information that we have. The vast majority are simply not ready to take that step. We are all chasing the small percentage of patients who are ready to make that decision and pay for that appointment up front.

This is leaving the other 90%+ with nobody to begin a relationship with them.

Instead, I recommend that you give them some useful information so that they can start to see the value in trusting your clinic. By doing this you will show that your clinic is different to all of your competitors clinics who fail to recognise that these potential patients have legitimate reservations.

Get the 90%+ who are not ready right now to slowly know, like and trust you and when they are ready to make a choice your clinic will be the obvious choice as yours was the clinic that offered assistance in advance while asking for nothing all so that you could help them on their journey to recovery.

It's my strong belief that it's time the podiatry profession began to reevaluate how we interact with the public who need our help and how we present ourselves to them. If we don't make this change, the Podiatry professional will continue to suffer a dramatic dropout rate. Owners of private podiatric things will continue to struggle with high levels of stress and we will continue to see other professions deliver poor care when it comes to foot problems.

The secret to running and scaling a successful Podiatry Practice is that clever marketing and a good quality marketing plan can help us to overcome our business problems.

When we recognise that we need to assist potential patient's fears and reservations when it comes to placing their trust in medical professionals like Podiatrists we will profit from it.

SECRET NO 8.

Always Use The Marketing Triad.

By now, hopefully you're starting to realise that the marketing that all those other clinics, your competitors, are doing is simply not going to deliver you and your clinic the quality or quantity of patient's needed to attain the financial and personal freedom you desire. It's not going to deliver you the life you hoped for when you quit that secure job, took a risk and opened your doors to patients.

It is my fervent wish that you now realise that you need to approach your marketing in a different way, a better way. An approach that gets your ideal patients to consider your clinic as the obvious choice before any of your competitors.

I'm also hoping that you realise the need for you to have a marketing plan that goes after your ideal patients like a heat seeking missile and a plan that holds your marketing spend fully accountable.

A lot of marketers will tell you that marketing is supposed to be an upfront loss. They will say that you should not expect to make your money back straight away.

Well, this is not how I like to do it. I like to at the very least break even, but more particularly, make a return on the spend my marketing spend straight away. For example, my Facebook marketing gives me a return of 15 to 1. My SMS reactivation campaign gives me a return of 16 to 1. My Newspaper ads give me a return of a minimum 4 to 1, sometimes 10 to 1 depending on the ad and where I run it.

At all points, I want to know how much I've spent and what return I get and I expect to make a profit straight away. You should be aiming to do the same to avoid any waste.

My budget and I suspect yours isn't as big as Coca Cola, or Budweiser, or those big brands. I don't have the money to spend on brand advertising or on loss making marketing.

In my own clinic, I sit down with my marketing manager in the middle of every single month and we plan out our marketing plan for the following month. To begin with, we look at the results from the previous month and hold that marketing spend accountable. We then use this information and any new plans we have to develop our marketing plan for the following month.

I consider my role is to help my marketing manager make sure that she has all of the tools, all of the resources, all of the training and the funding in place to carry out the marketing plan we have devised.

When we sit down together and develop our monthly marketing plan, we are at all times aware of the marketing triad.

So what is the marketing triad?

When I first start working with coaching clients, as part of my coaching program, I ask them what type of patients they treat and what type of patients would they prefer to treat? This usually confuses them, as they have been trained to treat anybody with a foot who comes in the door.

Now don't misunderstand me, in my own business we will not turn away too many patients from our clinic but to try and market or advertise to absolutely everybody who potentially could come into your clinic is a recipe for disaster.

This is too big of a pool of people for you and your clinic to market to effectively. What ends up happening when you take this scatter-gun approach is your marketing is completely diluted and the results are unreliable at best.

⊰○⊱

To ensure the best possible results from your marketing spend, you need to know 3 things

1st: Who is your ideal patient?

2nd: What message do you want to tell them?

3rd: What media do you need to use to get that message to your ideal patient?

Part one of your marketing triad: Your Ideal Patient.

It's not possible for you unless you are a multi million pound business to have a large enough marketing spend to cover all potential patients. Therefore, you must decide what is your ideal patient?

Now you have two ways to approach this. You can approach it by saying who is the ideal patient I'd like to treat or you can ask who is the ideal patient that will come in, be compliant with my treatment, is able to afford my treatment and will reach their goals.

I recently had a conversation like this with a coaching client of mine. Immediately when I asked him who his ideal patient was, he said, runners and triathletes. However, when we delved into it a bit deeper, he agreed that these patients only tend to come for one or two appointments as they want a quick fix.

These patients while they are happy to spend thousands on a new bike or new runners are not quite so happy to spend time and effort on their health and are more interested in getting back running as soon as possible, even if partially injured.

When we looked at the numbers we found that these patient's, while the injuries they had and the treatment was quite exciting, their profitability to the clinic was quite low. Instead, my client found that the type of patient he wanted to target to ensure the clinics financial and onward success would continue to grow were less exciting to treat but much more profitable.

Personally, I like to treat patients who turn up on time for their appointment, respect what I do, are compliant with their treatment, are able to and willing to pay for their treatment and get a good outcome. I'm happy to let the patients who want a quick fix, go to other clinics.

I target patients who I find easy to work with and are profitable to my clinic and I would suggest you do the same.

To this end, when I first started to laser focus my marketing, I decided that I would target a certain ideal patient. I like to call her Noreen. Noreen is a lady 50 - 65+ years old who is very compliant, is able to afford the treatment recommended and as a result gets a great outcome.

Below is my actual avatar for Noreen(my ideal patient) and you need to develop you Ideal Patient Avatar before you spend any money on any further marketing.

My Ideal Patient is "Noreen" 60 years old married to John for 35 yrs with 4 kids and 8 grandchildren who all live within 10 minutes of the house they grew up in and call over all the time for babysitting as much as anything. Noreen doesn't mind though because she lives for her family and things are harder now for her kids than in her time. John is close to retirement and is the main breadwinner.

Noreen works a few hours a week just to keep active but is thinking of stopping because she is slowing down and finding it harder to keep going, not that she's complaining because you young ones have it harder. John and her earn about €60,000 but paid the mortgage off years ago because the banks didn't give big loans out back then.

She's on Facebook and email, mainly to keep in touch with the kids, reads the local paper every single week and likes to listen to that controversial DJ on the local radio station.

She goes to Spain twice a year and loves to meet her friends(other Noreens) in town for coffee and go to Pennys and Marks & Spencers for a look. She meets her daughter in town on Saturday and takes the grand-kids for a walk but finds it harder to push the buggy because of her foot pain and is kind of happy when all the grand-kids go home and she and John can watch the soaps with a cup of tea.

Noreens has been having pain in her heel for the past 9 months which is not getting better even though she went to the gp and he gave her an injection. She is worried that she is getting older and can't do all the things she used to. Her daughters are telling her what to do and who to go see.

She doesn't know who to trust because she went to the doctor who said it's just her age and she already got insoles from "That Place In Town" which only fit in ugly shoes. She is worried she will have to wear "granny shoes" like the ones her mother used to wear at the end of her life when she didn't care about her appearance as much.

She doesn't want to run or anything but looks at Margaret next door who walks to town and back everyday since she went to that new clinic down the road. Noreen has looked them up on google and asked Margaret all about them but is not sure they can help her because that nice physio didn't fix her heel pain either.

She is very worried that she is going to get older and slower and be a burden on her daughters and afraid to spend any more money because John might give out again for wasting more money. She already has a box full of shoes and insoles hidden from John under the bed.

She just wishes someone would take the decision out of her hand and guarantee her that they could fix it whatever the price. She has decided to just wait and see if it goes rather than take any risks with more treatments.

You need to decide who the patient that you want to attract into your clinic is. Not just who's fun to treat, but who is going to be profitable to your clinic.

You need to know as much as you possibly can about your ideal patient.

- What activities does your idea patients do?

- What's their demographic?

- What's their family situation like?

- What hobbies do they like to do?

- Where do they live?

- Where do they hang out?

- Are they on Facebook or Instagram etc?

- Where do they get their news?

- What papers or magazines do they look at?

All of this information, the more detailed you can be, will mean that when you set up your marketing plan, it will be more laser focused resulting in less waste of your marketing budget and a greater return for the effort.

Part Two of the marketing triad; Your Message.

You need to be clear on what message you want to give to that ideal client. Your ideal client doesn't really care what your degree is in, what qualification you have, what fancy machines you have, what letters you have behind your name.

Your ideal client cares about what you can do for them. Why would they care about anything else?

You need to question your ideal client, find out what they want from your clinic not just what you want to give them. This will allow you to structure your message so that is it triggers a response from them, an emotional response, that encourages them to go ahead and begin the buying journey with your clinic.

Part 1 and Part 2 of the marketing triad are the most important part.

Knowing who your ideal client patient is, and what message will work with them is the most important parts of your marketing and you must get it right. If you don't invest time in these parts properly the result will be your marketing will be ineffective when you place this message in front of your ideal patient wherever they are and be unable to move them closer to making a decision to choose your clinic.

Part 3 of The Marketing Triad; The Media You Use.

One of the biggest mistakes I see that most businesses, including Podiatry clinics, make is they start with the media. They assume that because everybody is on the latest media, such as Facebook or Instagram that they should be active on it too.

I ask you what's the point in being on Facebook or Instagram if your ideal client isn't there? This is why you have to come up with your detailed avatar. So my ideal client, as I said, is Noreen, who is 50 to 65+. Noreen is not on Twitter nor is she on Instagram, hence, I don't use any of my marketing spend on Twitter or Instagram. Noreen hangs out on Facebook. Noreen reads the local newspaper which is free, which is why I do newspaper advertising in that paper only.

Don't make the mistake of starting at the end, the media. Don't do what your competitors are doing, spending their marketing budget in Google Ads or Facebook and not stopping to think who they are trying to talk to and what they need to say to them to make that connection.

So to recap, you have the three parts of the marketing triad;

1. **Our ideal patient or avatar**

2. **The message we want to send them**

3. **The media we use it in.**

An example of how this works is my ideal client, a lady as I said, 55-65+ who has sore feet and is unable to exercise as much as her husband. She feels she's getting old, has been to a number of other clinics, has spent a lot of money and is disappointed with the results and now has a pair of orthotics that she can't fit into any shoes other than her runners.

We know that this ideal client hangs out on Facebook, as the largest growing demographic on Facebook is ladies 60+, therefore we meet that ideal patient on Facebook with the message asking her is she having problems with her feet?

Is she finding that she's got orthotics that are disappointing her or had treatment elsewhere spending money with little or no results.

Now I understand that this will not trigger results with all ladies over 50-65yrs+, but I don't want all ladies 50-65yrs+. I only want those ladies with sore feet who who feel the message that I am putting in front of them speaks to them, as these are my ideal patient.

This will encourage them to move to the next step on my marketing funnel, my website where they will find free information upfront (that we discussed in the Secret 7) which they will get in exchange for contact details, allowing me to follow up with them.

This targeting allows me to keep my marketing spend lower than I would otherwise have had to do to get the same results and gives me more bang for my buck.

An example of how NOT TO DO THIS, a number of years ago when I ran a newspaper advertisement in a local Free newspaper that was primarily read by adults who were 65 +. This paper was read by my ideal client and had given great results in the past. I was given big discount so placed a half page advertisement offering Free Running Injury Assessments in a rush.

Well guess what? The people reading the paper were not running so I got ZERO response to the advertisement. I had wasted €300 on an ad because I hadn't taken the time to think?

Yes, I knew who I wanted to target. My message was really good and my ad copy was very very good. My mistake was I had placed it somewhere that the avatar the ad was built for, a runner, would not be found as they did not read this paper.

I hope you can now see how the marketing triad is the key to any marketing decisions that you do. Otherwise, you're just throwing money out there and hoping that some of it hits the jackpot. This is how most small businesses never mind most podiatry clinics do their business. It's a blind fishing expedition.

If you wanted a big fish you would first figure what fish type to target, what bait they respond to and finally where to find them.

So far in this Secret No 8 and Secret No 7 before, we've laid all the groundwork for marketing, we figured out what not to do, who to target, what message to give them and where to find them. In Secrets Nos 9 & 10, we will start to discuss how we implement this marketing.

We begin with internal marketing, as it's much cheaper and quicker to get up and running. I will then move on to external marketing, which is what everybody wants to do straight away when they first become a client of mine as they think more new patient's is the answer to all of their clinics troubles and probably what you may be thinking.

The secret to having Podiatry clinic that gives you more freedom while earning more is using the Marketing Triad in all of your clinics marketing.

SECRET NO 9.

Start With Internal Marketing, It's Simpler By Far

If you are just getting started with marketing, or realise that maybe you need to restart your marketing, then I suggest that you begin with internal marketing.

Internal marketing is any sort of marketing that you do to the patient's that you already have within your clinic. These are patients that.

You have already built a relationship with and who know your clinic. They know your culture and have had an opportunity to like and trust you and your clinic. These patients are far more inclined to buy services from you again. We tend to buy from people we like and as these patients already know and hopefully like you they will buy again.

Depending on what research you read, you will find various numbers stating that it costs between 10 and 14 times more to get a brand new customer/patient than it does to get a previous customer/patient to come back and buy again. Think about the last time you decided to go on a night out and you were deciding which restaurant to go to. The first thing to pop into your mind would be the last one or two restaurants you had been to that you'd had a great experience. It's far more likely that you would have chosen these restaurants, than gone online and picked another restaurant you didn't know and weren't too sure whether you could trust to have the same experience.

Marketing internally to the patients you already have on your books to either get them to spend more on other services you offer, come more often or return after a break from your clinic is the simplest and cheapest way for you to boost your profits while delivering great quality ethical care to your patients.

I'll give you two examples:

Example 1. I run a fully automated SMS reactivation system in my own clinic and I help my coaching clients to set up systems like this in their clinics. This system sends automated SMS messages to my patients at predetermined intervals. This can be designed to send different types of messages to the different types of patients be they a Chiropody appointment, a biomechanical issue and so forth checking in to see how these patients are getting on since they were last in.

In all cases, these SMS reactivation texts are primarily following up on our patients to make sure that they are still achieving the goals that they wanted to. At the time of writing this book, this is giving a return on investment of approximately

16 to 1. What this means is, for every €1 that is spent on this internal marketing system, which is fully automated, we make a return of €16. This internal marketing system works 24/7, 365 days a year, even while I'm on holiday.

Example number 2. I recently started to work with a podiatrist who had been in business for a number of years. He had never measured the number of patients who would return for a second appointment, just assuming that they would do so if he suggested it. When we started to measure this accurately using a software system, he was stunned to see that out of 100 patients he would see, only 17% were booking a follow up appointment. He freely admitted that it was highly unlikely that he was fixing the complex cases he was seeing in one single appointment.

We set about working on this and improving his rebooking system. This internal marketing whereby he would encourage his patient to book that second appointment resulted in a 14 day turnaround of a 17% rebooking rate improving to a 65% rebooking rate. This simple internal marketing system led to an approximate 56% increase in this podiatrists turnover in less than a 6 months period without any additional external marketing spend.

When you have a limited budget for marketing, the easiest way to begin is to begin with your internal marketing. Make the most of the resources you have by helping the patients that you already have on your books. Obviously, I'm not suggesting that you ever sell them a service they do not need. This would go against every fibre of my being and I'm sure yours. However, internal marketing allows you to ethically help your existing patients get the best quality care from a clinic, your clinic, that they already know, they already trust and they already like.

Both of the examples I have demonstrated above clearly demonstrate the power of internal marketing. Internal marketing is not only much cheaper to run than acquiring new patients, but usually requires much less work to set up and helps to build a more loyal patient database as you cement the relationship that you have with them.

There are lots of other ways to get patients you've already helped to use more of your services, ie; Internal Marketing examples.

Welcome Letter.

Every new patient that comes to my clinic receives a welcome letter in the post within 24 to 48 hours. This is a physical letter, signed by me, which thanks them for coming to see us. It explains to them the clinics story, who the staff members are and how, by deciding to choose my clinic whose livelihoods they are supporting. Why do I do this? Well it puts a human dimension on their choice of where they spend their hard earned money. In with this letter is an upsell letter. This upsell letter is a simple sheet explaining all of the other services we do and attached to this are 2 referral vouchers that they can give to friends or loved ones to a Free Assessments.

This achieves two things. Firstly, a patient may come in with a corn, not realising that we also treat plantar fasciitis or knee pain. When they get the welcome letter, they are made aware that we do so. They might also find that it's their spouse who has heel pain and now in possession of the free assessment voucher they could pass that on to their spouse and suggest they go and visit this nice clinic that they've been to.

This internal marketing welcome letter is extremely simple and very cheap to run.

I have included a sample of in the bonus section for this book @

www.morepracticeprofits.com/podiatry-business-book-bonus

Broadcast email.

A Broadcast email is an email that is sent to your patient database at regular intervals, I do it weekly. The important thing is to send it at regular intervals so that your patients know when to expect it. The broadcast email should be full of useful information that your patients look forward to reading.

It should begin with friendly insights into you the clinicians life. Again, this helps your patient's to get to know, like and trust you and break down the barrier of you and your clinic just being the usual unemotional purely professional clinic that develops minimal patient loyalty. The patient who feels they know you somewhat personally is more likely to stay loyal to you and your clinic and is more likely to recommend you to their friends and loved ones.

As part of the broadcast email, I like to add a section on our weekly blog, which, in turn, helps our SEO marketing. Finally and probably most importantly, in the P.S .section, I'd like to add an offer. I don't give an offer every single time I send a broadcast email, as I don't want the email to come across as purely a sales message. It needs to be something that the patient feels it's got something in it for them, useful friendly information with a soft sell on occasion.

Usually for every four broadcast emails that I send weekly, one of them will have a soft offer, such as 50% off some new procedure that we've started. As your patients get used to the idea of the broadcast email coming in you can always be used as a supplementary way to boost your diary if you're having a quiet week.

For example, last year, I took on a new member of staff, a physical therapist and it had been a while since we last had one. So naturally, there was little or no work for him when he started. He was due to start on Monday and the previous

Wednesday we had sent out a broadcast email with an offer of 75% off an initial assessment with him for Back Pain.

The first week he started his book was full and of these 80% booked in for a full plan of care, filling his first month in advance within 5 days and boosting the clinic's profit for the next two to three months. If I was to use external marketing to get the same result it would have taken weeks if not months to do the same and the cost of this email was pennies at most. In fact broadcast email can be used very simply with email systems such as MailChimp which begin at a cost of free.

I have included a sample Broadcast Email in the bonus section for this book @

www.morepracticeprofits.com/podiatry-business-book-bonus

Referral Reward.

Word of mouth is a huge part of any podiatry clinic and for most clinics, that have little or no marketing planning, it is the main part of their marketing. It's how they find most of their patients. It is how most podiatry clinics develop a new patient base. Unfortunately, most of these same clinics have no system to encourage this word of mouth referral process.

A referral reward system is quite easy to set up and will encourage your patients who already know, like and trust you to recommend you to their family and friends. You might say, well, they already do that and that's probably true. However, studies show that the longer it's been since a customer or patient in your case has partaken of your services, the less likely they are to remember the good quality service and recommend you to others.

You need to be able to remind them or encourage them to continue to recommend you long after they finished treatment with your clinic. You should aim to turn them into raving fans of your clinic that cannot help but tell everyone to make sure they use you. This can be done in a number of ways.

To begin with, you should make sure that your patients know that you run a referral reward system. This in our clinic we do with signage in the clinic, with our welcome letter and in our broadcast email sequence. Once a new patient comes in and tells you who sent them, assuming you ask in the first place *(you should be asking)* you will then send that person a referral reward.

This can be done in the form of a simple thank you card with a reward inside the envelope. Rewards in my clinic have included a voucher for a bottle of wine and lunch in a local cafe. For the ladies, having a pedicure, or a manicure or cheaper again and highly effective is a voucher for a free appointment in your own clinic.

We send these in a gold envelope with a handwritten address on the front. This will encourage the recipient to open this letter before any others with excitement of finding out what's inside the gold envelope. Once they open it, they find a letter signed by myself thanking them for the referral with a voucher on a golden ticket included, just like in Charlie's Chocolate Factory.

You can test the rewards that you use to see which is most effective in your area. The important thing is that by doing this, you are saying thank you to previous patients who are sending you new patients and encouraging them to continue that process.

Think about the last time you recommended someone to a local business. Did the business ever call you and say thank you. I doubt it. If they had, would it have made you more likely to do the same thing? I suspect it would.

Upsell Letters.

When I talk about upsell letters, I am of course not suggesting that you would ever sell or recommend any sort of treatment or service that is inappropriate. However, lots of patients that come to your clinic are likely not fully aware of the range of services that you can provide them. I remember a number of years ago when I had a particular physiotherapist working for me he was treating a lady whose ankle was troublesome, having been given the referral from my podiatry team. She was on her fourth appointment in the clinic and informed the physiotherapist that she needed to go and find a physio clinic as she also had a problem with her back. She was not aware that he could also treat her back. This is where an upsell letter would come in and make sure that a patient like this lady was fully aware of all the services she could get in the clinic including those she did not initially attend for.

A simple letter that you will give to your patient, either in physical form through the post, or by email explaining to them all of the services that you provide will suffice. This could be done when the patient arrives initially and has to fill a new patient form and read your terms and conditions. It can also be done when you send them the welcome letter, as we do in our clinic, explaining to them all of the other services that you do and a voucher to try out one of those services.

During your broadcast email, you have an opportunity to explain to patients any new services that you may be providing or alternative services that they haven't had before. All of this can be streamed depending on the type of appointment that that patient had initially.

For example, a patient who had attended for a chiropody appointment might be advised that you also treat Heel Pain or vice versa. A mother who brought her child in for an ingrown toenail might also be informed that we treat her older child's verruca.

These upsell letters can be developed well in advance and used daily with all new and current patients.

Reactivation of Past Patients

Unless you're a brand new clinic, you will have a database of patients who have been to you before hopefully all of whom were happy with the treatment. It's a matter of fact, that not all of these will continue to come back to you long term. Some may have moved away, some may unfortunately have passed away, but others may have simply forgotten that you exist.

This is an opportunity for you to reactivate those patients and have them return to your clinic at very reduced cost to you. How you do so is less important but it can be done either by email, direct mail, or my favourite SMS automated system. Simply by checking in with these patients after a set period of time on how they're progressing it is possible to reactivate that patient and have them return to your clinic.

A favourite of mine is a free 12 month orthotic checkup. Any patient who has received orthotics will get a letter in the post, offering them a free checkup of their orthotics 12 months on. I find that a lot of those patients who will return have perhaps a minor issue that needs some assistance and in a lot of cases, they request a repeat pair of orthotics.

This, like I said, can be automated if you have a good CRM system. In our case, we combine *Cliniko* with *Cliniqapps* to do this and follow it up with a physical letter.

Reactivation of your current database of past patients is the simplest and cheapest way for you to boost your turnover, while providing good quality care to people who already have tried your clinic and know like and trust you. Once these patients are reactivated, you can then encourage them to refer their friends and family. This then can become an exponential growth process.

Signage In The Clinic.

Most clinics will have signs somewhere in their clinic. However, usually the signs are not particularly pleasant, such as, *"don't ask for credit"* or *"cheques must be made out to...."* . These are not the friendliest welcome to give patient's and instead you should consider replacing them with messages of the services that you do and offers that you're providing.

I would recommend that you procure yourself a number of signage frames that allow you to change the sign routinely. This should be placed in all of your clinics and in the waiting room, even in the bathroom, with an offer of the week or offer of the month. In my own clinic we replace these every two weeks with a new offer.

An example of which can be found at bonus for purchasers or this book at

www.morepracticeprofits.com/podiatry-business-book-bonus

We have we have 13 of these signs which we rotate twice a year. All of these should be done tastefully and offer attractive options such as a free child's foot assessment or 50% off orthotic refurbishment to patient's.

Start to replace any unattractive or unfriendly signage with more effective internal signage, you can develop quite cheaply on sites such as *vistaprint.com* etc , to encourage your current patients to avail of more services,

Phone Waiting Systems.

Nowadays it's quite simple, especially with ISDN lines to set up messages while patients are waiting on the phone. These messages can explain your services or your offer of the month and as with the signage in the clinic, can be rotated on a regular basis.

Cancellation & DNA Calls.

We like to ring patients who have cancelled without a follow up appointment made or those who have not attended a scheduled appointment. The primary reason for doing this is to check in and make sure that they're okay.

A bonus with these calls is in a lot of cases, those patients have not reached 100% of where they wanted to get to and have had to put off the appointment.

I understand that life gets in the way of a patient's best intentions. However, following a conversation with my clinical team, when appropriate, we would encourage the patient to rebook that appointment or we would put it into our diary to follow up with them again, after an agreed time to organize that cancelled appointment. This is done to make sure that patient reaches the health goal that they stipulated to us on their initial appointment.

Letters To Other Medics Who Refer.

Like word of mouth, a large part of referral system for most podiatry clinics that are starting out or have little to no marketing is referrals from other medics such as GP's. It is vital that you return a thank you letter explaining what you have done with their patient.

Doing this encourages that physician to trust your medical abilities and makes it far more likely that they will recommend to the next patient that is suitable for your clinic that they attend your clinic.

These letters do not need to be very long or detailed. Your local GP is receiving hundreds of letters a month and does not have time to read an encyclopedic description of your case history. A simple letter thanking them for the referral, explaining what the diagnosis is and what your treatment plan is enough. Perhaps send another one further down the line once you have fixed the patient telling the referrer that you have resolved the patient's issue will give them confidence that you are looking after their patients as they would wish.

I hope by now you can see the internal marketing is where you should start when you decide to develop your marketing plan. It's much cheaper, much simpler to do and will take less of your time to get set up and organise than external marketing. You already have a database of patients and you should focus on continuing to develop these relationships as well as you possibly can before you start to encourage more new clients to come in the door.

If you have limited budget to spend on your marketing, you're better off to begin spending it on your internal marketing system. This is what I do with all of my coaching clients.

Obviously, we all want to begin with the nice shiny object which is external marketing, such as Facebook and Google and so forth but your internal marketing is where the low hanging fruit are. Start with your internal marketing system and once you have it running really well only then start with your external marketing.

Think of it as a leaky bucket. If you have a bucket full of holes, and all of your current patients are dropping out down the bottom, turning the tap on and filling that bucket with more water is just simply wasting your money.

The secret to having a profitable podiatry practice is to have a slick internal marketing system.

SECRET NO 10.

Rock Your Podiatry Clinic With Amazing External Marketing

What exactly is external marketing anyway? How is different to internal marketing?

External marketing is any marketing you do external to your Podiatry clinic in an effort to gain new patients. It should not be confused with internal marketing to current or past patients.

External marketing is what most clinic owners think of when they think of marketing. They think Facebook, Google, the newspaper, Yellow pages and so forth, but in truth this is just external marketing, not the whole of marketing.

External marketing is much much more expensive and it's much harder to pull off than internal marketing.

Why is this?

The reason for this is because you are trying to convince people who have no idea who you are that they should trust you above all of your competitors.

How Do Your Potential Patients Decide Which Clinic To Choose?

You are trying to convince them that they should trust you with their health. You are trying to convince them that they should trust you with their hard earned money. They don't know you from all the other clinics in town. They don't understand that you are "better" than all those other clinics and that you "care more", that you've been on more courses and that you studied harder than your competitors.

Frankly, they don't care. All they care about is can you fix them and how can you guarantee them that you can do so. Imagine for a moment that you need a service.

For example, you have a leak in your house and you need a plumber. What you're most likely to do is to take out your smartphone, search for a "plumber near me" or the name of the town that you're in. Depending on how good the plumber is at marketing he may or he may not show up on the first page. If he does, he might be at the top but there might be others before him, depending on how tuned in he is to his marketing.

This is how most of us find a service nowadays when we're actively looking for it and unless you know what you're doing it's a lottery whether you get picked or not. This plumber may or may not be cultivating reviews on Google. He may or may not have a *Google My Business Page* setup and know what he is doing with regards to it. Most clinic owners have no clue how to do this.

Or imagine for a moment that you're looking to book something that you've been researching for quite a while, such as a long family holiday that you've been looking forward to for the last two years. Perhaps you decided to take yourself and your family to Bali for two weeks and you're not just going to pick the first one that comes along. It's quite likely you'll do an awful lot of research online. You will look at the reviews of places you are considering going to. You might get quotes from a number of different sites before you make a decision.

Your potential and future patient's are doing the same thing right now as you read this line. They are checking out your clinic and your competitors clinics at home on the couch with their smartphones.

The online world has made it possible for smart clinics to scale up their clinic exponentially but if you don't know what you're doing you can waste most of your marketing budget on ineffective advertising. Getting new customers to choose you over all of those other options they have is a tough gig.

The Mistakes I See With External Marketing of Podiatry Clinics.

What I find most clinic owners do is they'll have an ad in the yellow pages and they quite likely will have a Facebook page. Often they will copy other local clinics or businesses, perhaps running a small promotion to get people to like or share their Facebook page thinking this will lead to increased income. Well, likes on your Facebook page is simply not effective marketing, you can't bring a Facebook share to the bank.

Did you know that Facebook will not show 100% of the people that like your page all of your posts, instead only showing only 2-5% of them. Sometimes the clinic owner may have posts on Twitter or Instagram even if their ideal patient's are not on Twitter or Instagram. They might do the odd newspaper ad if the newspapers salesman asks.

A clinic close to mine has ad in a newspaper every single week that's simply lists the name of the owner all of their initials, phone number and a "Book Now" call to action. This is hardly a compelling reason to pick up the phone and ring them but they're spending hundreds of Euros every single year on this crappy ad.

Almost every single podiatric clinic I look at has a pretty but basic brochure website which does little or nothing to encourage patients to come in. It doesn't doesn't differentiate them from their competitors and it's usually set up once and left alone with the owner assuming that this will lead to patients choosing their clinic over all others, even though the websites are all saying the same thing.

The truth is that most clinics hope that their local doctors or some other medics will refer some patients to them but they have no system for cultivating these word of mouth referrals.

External Marketing Mistakes Lead To Stagnation.

I have made all of these mistakes myself and the result was stagnation.

On the outside the clinic seemed to be quite busy and we had a great name with the local medical community. However joe public had no idea who I was, or whether they should choose my clinic over my competitors some of whom had done their training course on the internet.

It retrospect I realise now that the public couldn't have known any different when my website didn't speak to them. It was all about me and not about them and their worries. In fact, my whole marketing was all about me and nothing to do with the patient and what they would be looking for.

Nowadays of course I've wised up and I have a highly automated marketing system that makes my ideal patients choose my clinic before my competitors. My mostly automated external marketing system makes my clinic the obvious choice. The longer I am running the system the cheaper it is becoming for me to get the same type of new patients to pick up the phone to us. When I do get this new patient, they then go into my internal marketing and my reactivation marketing systems.

Isn't Doctor Referrals Going To Be Enough?

Like I said earlier, most podiatry clinics go straight to their local doctors and hope that they will send them some patients. We still have good relationships with the local medics, but I find they're just not dependable. They may retire, they may forget who you are or a new podiatry clinic may open down the road and they might decide that they will refer there for a change. Perhaps they'll decide that they're going to do some of the treatments themselves that they used to refer to you for.

While I have great respect for the local medics, I do not depend on them for my livelihood and I don't think you should either. The answer is to bypass your doctor and go straight for your ideal patient. This is why it's so important that you know your avatar or ideal client. If you don't know who you're targeting, how are you supposed to target them efficiently and not waste your marketing budget on people who were never suitable for your clinic to begin with.

The strategy that I have my clients in my coaching program perform is to get potential patients into their marketing funnel by going to where their potential patients are hanging out. That may be Google, Facebook and so on and then offering those ideal clients, upfront, useful information for free in exchange for their contact details. They then follow up with these patients relentlessly, thus building a relationship, using a combination of email, phone calls, direct mail, information, events, etc.

Those potential patients or ideal client, get to know, like and trust your clinic as a result of this. When they are ready to make a decision on who they're going to get to help them with their foot pain, there is one obvious choice that they're going to make..... the clinic that was happy to put their hand out and help them in advance of asking for money.

Automate Your External Marketing So It Works When You Don't.

As I mentioned earlier, this can be highly automated. Software systems like *Infusionsoft, Kajabi* are all singing all dancing and I have used both. While these systems are expensive, they have paid for themselves over and over again. You can use more simplistic versions like *Drip, ClickFunnels* and even *MailChimp*.

The software systems can be used in varying degrees of complexity. Depending on the software you pick you can set them up to automate emails to ideal clients, staff, phone calls, letters and even SMS.

The Fortune Is In The Follow Up.

The key here is that you continue to follow up with your ideal client. A mentor of mine once told me the fortune is in the follow up. What we do in my clinic and I have my clients do is what most clinic owners don't do........we follow up relentlessly. I instruct my staff to follow up with the patient until either they have booked an appointment or they ask us not to follow up with them anymore.

Now you might say this is not what the patient wants. The common response I get from clinic owners is *"Lorcan the patient will not want us continually phoning up asking them to book an appointment"*. These clinic owners are 100% right, but this is not what we do.

When my team follow up, we continually give more and more useful information to help them make a decision on how they can resolve their issue, even if we suggest the best choice is going to another clinic. The result is 70% of patients who enter our funnel *(cold leads to begin with mind you)* book an appointment with us.

With this system it's possible for us to turn up or down like a dial the inflow into the funnel with the ability to predict how many of those patients will book an appointment and proceed with care.

How good would it be to have a marketing tap that you could turn up and down as you need it in your clinic?

The Follow Up Phone Call.

While we do follow up with email, direct mail and SMS, the key in the early stages of this follow up system is the phone call. This is done as soon as possible after the patient has taken that initial step and giving you their contact details. Remember, you need to take the approach that you're giving useful information for free in advance.

I will give you an example:

Just today as I write this, its Monday afternoon and over the weekend we had a lady download a free report off our website on how to help her plantar fascia pain. She was given a call by my admin team this morning at 10 o'clock to see had she been able to download the report. Once the discussion was started, we asked her how she'd been getting on.

She told us that she had been having pain for the past four to six weeks and hadn't had any treatment. We gave her some advice about what she could consider doing at home and told her that we would give her a call in another 5-7 days to see how she got on with the useful tips inside the report. Now, it's not likely that this patient will be able to resolve her pain completely on her own. If she does that's great as we will have gained another fan. However, if in 7 days time when we give her another call, she has not resolved her issue, it is more likely that she will pick us as the clinic to help get rid herself of her pain.

The key to the phone call is to encourage your patient to tell their story. It allows them to build trust in you and your clinics abilities. The longer you spend on the phone, the more likely they are to go ahead and choose you as a clinic. I advise my coaching clients to spend at least 10 minutes on the phone with the patient. The motto we have is.... *"keep the conversation going".* This might be over one call or multiple calls and when that patient is ready, we make them an offer.

What To Offer Them To Get Them To Come In Your Door That 1st Time.

We have a number of offers that we may utilise depending on how far we think the potential patient is along the journey to making a choice. Firstly we may offer them a free or paid appointment. If we feel are not ready for a paid appointment, to reduce scepticism we will offer them a Free Foot assessment.

In a free foot assessment the potential patient will get to come in and meet one of my podiatry team for 20 to 30 minutes at absolutely no charge. They are made aware that this will be an information only appointment where the podiatrists will give them a differential diagnosis and an idea of what they should expect is going to be needed to be able to resolve it, what their next step is and the cost of that next appointment.

These free consults are very popular with patients who are sceptical because they've usually had treatment elsewhere and been disappointed by their treatment.

However, some patients are even too sceptical for this, so we may offer them a free follow up call with one of the podiatry team over the phone or a follow up call one of the admin team depending on who has developed the best rapport with the patient.

Don't Think You Have To Sacrifice Your Moral Code.

As I said earlier, we find seven of the 10 of these patients end up in a treatment plan in our clinic. In all cases, the information and advice we give them is best practice and is appropriate to their care. If we have a patient that comes in for a free appointment and no treatment is necessary they will be advised of this. Just because you're marketing and trying to get patients to come to see does not mean that you have to sacrifice your ethical or moral code.

Your patient is looking for solutions. I believe it is our responsibility as medics to present them with all of the options for them to achieve this solution. Hiding away in your clinic and not presenting your ability to help that patient could be argued to be unethical. That patient may make the wrong decision and get the wrong treatment. I'm sure you can think of patients who have come to you who have had treatment elsewhere that you knew was completely incorrect or inappropriate and you wished they had just come to see you before they went elsewhere.

Remember the key to external marketing is as I said is you need to know your ideal patient inside out.....

You need to know as much as you possibly can about them, what their fears are, what their hopes are, where they hang out, what they do all day.

You need to recognise their scepticism and what has happened to them in the past.

You then need to be able to target where they are in their patient journey.

You should be willing and able to provide them with useful information, in advance of any payment, in exchange for their contact details.

They should be entered into your marketing funnel, which has been set up in advance and you need to follow up, follow up and follow up some more, at all stages, providing them with useful information that allows them to come to the right decision with regards to their healthcare,

By being empathetic with the patient, understanding their scepticism and giving help upfront in advance of any payment and you will reap the rewards just as I have done and my coaching clients continue to do. Empathy and caring are not the same thing. Empathy has to learned and consciously practised.

Filling Your Marketing Funnel

The following section is about different ways to get your patient or your ideal client into your marketing funnel so you and your team can follow up with them. This is where most clinic owners tend to get bogged down.

Remember our marketing triad where we had "your market" or your ideal client, "your message", what you want to tell them and "your media", what media you are going to use to deliver your message to your ideal client.

What most podiatry clinic owners do is they start with the media. They start with Facebook, they go straight to Google ads or they build a website but they have no idea what they want to say or who they want to say it to. I have seen clinic owners being very active on Twitter with blogs and information that is targeted towards patients who are not even on Twitter. It is a complete waste of their time. They have not thought out in advance what they're doing.

We as clinic owners tend to get blinded by the latest shiny social media we feel we should be on. These are just tools to use, not necessarily a guarantee of success. If you don't have your marketing message and know who you want to put this message in front of correct first you are setting yourself up for failure and wasted marketing budget.

However, your media does matter if your message is done correctly and if you know who your ideal client is and if you're delivering it in the right place to them (even if your copy isn't great) you are ahead of your competitors. There is a long list of various media that you can use to target your patients or ideal client

Google Ads.

Google ads, or Google AdWords is a mammoth in the field of marketing. Before the advent of the Internet, and the smartphone, if you wanted a local service, you took out your copy of the yellow pages and you would search alphabetically for that service. This was so important that when I first started my clinic in 2005 I like most people wanted to be at the top of the page when it came to podiatrists. To do this I made sure my clinic began with an A hence I called my Achilles Foot Clinic.

Nowadays, I wouldn't do this and would instead, in all likelihood, call the clinic something to do with its location. People no longer pick up the phone book but instead they take out their smartphones. They type in the service they want, and the location that they wanted it in. Depending on what country you're in, you might take the area first, or the service first.

Certainly outside of the United States, and even within the United States, Google is king. If you're not on Google AdWords you're missing a trick, an open goal, to boost your marketing and your new patient numbers. The thing about Google is that when people go on to Google they are actively looking for a solution to their problem. They will type in their problem and Google will present them with a number of solutions or options.

It's imperative that you make sure that your podiatry clinic is presented to them first and foremost and in a way that encourages them to choose your ad before your competitors. Google Ads is a complex beast for newbies, you have to know how to devise your ad, your budget and the location you want it to run your ads. You have to make sure that the keywords you pick are effective. Are you choosing the correct negative keywords? I made the mistake for years of have no negative keywords and I was as a result bidding against myself!

Once you get this part right you need to make sure that the landing page that you send them to is working correctly by converting your leads into potential patients that will end up inside your marketing funnels. If you're sending your patients to your homepage you are making a big mistake and let's face it, this is what most podiatry clinics are doing. Start to develop specific landing pages and let your competitors keep making mistakes.

For years, I used Google ads, and was never sure of the return. However, a number of years ago, I decided I was going to get serious on it and I started to study it properly, got some expert help which I pay handsomely for. I now spend thousands a year on Google Ads and receive in return hundreds of thousands in directly attributable turnover.

Google AdWords has the capacity to change your clinic and boost your turnover like no other marketing can if done correctly. The imperative with Google Ads is not to spread yourself too thinly.

Consider running condition specific or location specific, or a combination of both, be sure your ads are designed with a targeted number of keywords which directly match the ads you are running and transfer your potential patient to a landing page that specifically deals with the search query that they have inputted into their smartphone.

For example, a patient who searches for verruca needs to see an ad that speaks about verruca. Not an ad that speaks about podiatry, or foot clinic. When they click on that ad you need to make sure that the landing page they arrive at is not your homepage, but rather a specifically designed landing page that speaks to them about their verruca and the solutions that you have for them.

That landing page should then offer them useful information on Verruca up front in exchange for their contact details, so that they automatically enter into your Verruca follow up system or marketing funnel.

This is the beauty of Google ads. It can work 24/7 for you while you're on holidays or even while you're asleep.

On the 2nd January this year when we opened our clinic, having been closed for two weeks, we had 50+ new leads waiting for us that Google Ads provided over the closed period.

How many of my competitors were able to open their doors at 8am on the 2nd January and have 50+ potential patients waiting for them to ring and start the conversation about why they were the best clinic to help them reach their goals. All this was possible using Google ads. While I sat on the couch watching Christmas movies and eating too many chocolates Google Ads was working for my business filling my diary.

Google Remarketing

Google also allows you to use its Google remarketing system. Google remarketing system is a retargeting system, whereby you have the ability to place code from Google on your website, which will result in anyone who lands on your website, having the ad for your clinic appear on their computer, smartphone, tablet etc even when they're not on your clinics website.

It is this system that other businesses use to remind you of purchases you were considering, maybe yesterday or last week. How else do you think that that website that you were looking at last week is now popping up all over the place on your smartphone. You too can use this in your clinic.

However you should note that Google does have strict rules with regards to its use for health clinics versus more normal retail businesses.

Google My Business.

Google My Business is a free service that Google allows you to claim showing past current and potential patients, your location, your website, your opening hours, your services, and so forth. It's important that you claim your Google My Business and that you begin to develop its content, including your Google reviews as activity here will be rewarded with regard to your SEO.

Google reviews is an easy way for potential patients to gain trust in your clinics abilities by seeing how people just like them got on when they used your services. This social proof or testimonials can be encouraged and is done so in my clinic in an automated fashion using SMS, email and direct mail.

This has led to a situation where we have 20 times more reviews than our nearest competitor has. All of which helps to build trust in the eyes of any potential patient when they're making a decision on which clinic will they will use for their treatment.

Facebook

Facebook advertising is a must if you wish to scale up your podiatry clinic. Facebook is the largest social media site on the planet by a mile. It has over 2 billion, read that again billion with a B, active users every month and over 1.5 billion daily users. These are people who are on almost all cases on Facebook on their mobile phone for a minimum of an average of 20 minutes. What I like about Facebook is it is fantastic for the ability to be able to zero in on your ideal patient or client.

Facebook marketing allows you to be very specific when it comes to demographics. You can choose the age profile, the sex, the interests, the area, etc. So for example, if you want to only advertise to male runners between the age of 35 and 45 in a 15 mile radius who are members of a certain Facebook group or browse a lot of running pages, Facebook will let you do this. Therefore, your advertising spend is not wasted on people who do not fit into this category. It is relatively cheap versus other forms of marketing.

However, you must remember that when you advertise on Facebook, people browsing Facebook are not actively looking for your service in the main. You are almost in all cases interrupting them from their browsing. They may or may not have any interest in what you have to say. Therefore, you need to approach your potential patient or prospect assuming that they are more sceptical than those who were perhaps using Google and that they are far less ready to book an appointment with you.

You should be offering free useful information or entertainment, such as quizzes etc and which we have been quite successful recently on Facebook. Also working well on Facebook at the moment are videos. It's important if you're doing a video that you should consider having text overlying it as a lot of people like to have the videos on mute on Facebook. This can be done quite simply through web sites like *fiverr. com* and *upwork.com*.

Another bonus of Facebook is the Facebook pixel. Facebook pixel is a piece of code that you put on your website which allows you to re-target visitors to your website through their Facebook feed.

Also of note is Facebook's rules when it comes to health care. They're pretty strict on not allowing you to suggest to your potential client that they may in any way have ill health. For example, your headline cannot say, *"Do you have sore feet?"* but it can say *"Sore feet clinic available now"*.

Facebook Groups

I'm sure we all know about Facebook groups. Most of us are members of Facebook groups professionally and otherwise. For example, I'm a member of the of both the UK Podiatry and the Ireland Podiatry Facebook groups and find them very useful.

Have you ever considered setting up a Facebook group for your patients? You could think of it like a VIP member group for your patients to contact the clinic. This can give the impression of exclusivity for your patients, as only members are admitted to the group.

Facebook Messenger etc...

Facebook Messenger should also be incorporated into your marketing plan as you should consider that your potential patient may have come across your ad on Facebook and wishes to message you straight away. The obvious way for them to do this is Facebook Messenger.

Lastly, you can add in a *Book Online* and a *Call Now* button or call to action on your clinics Facebook page. Give your patients the opportunity to go ahead with the choice that they are considering straight away such as booking online or calling straight away.

However, remember, when it comes to your ads on Facebook, this is not the approach you should be taking. You should take a more subtle long term approach to the advertising that you use in this media.

Instagram.

Instagram is owned by Facebook and it's relatively straightforward to set up an ad campaign on Instagram if you already are running a Facebook campaign. What you must remember about Instagram, is that although it has 1 billion active monthly users, and 500 million of these users daily, most of them are under the age of 35.

Instagram is the highest used social media for teenagers, higher even than Snapchat so before investing time and energy advertising on Instagram be sure the patient you are targeting is actually on it. On average users of Instagram spend longer on it than they do on Facebook. Instagram is primarily a visual media, one in which you need to be telling a story. Videos are very popular on Instagram.

Twitter.

Twitter has over 300 million monthly users and over 125 million daily active users. It's quite simple to use Twitter and if you include links in your Twitter feed, you will tend to get a greater response from your tweets.

I personally have never found any great success from the use of Twitter as I have found that my ideal patient is just not on twitter in any great numbers, so I tend not to spend any of my advertising budget on it. However, this may not be the case for you. It will entirely depend on who your ideal patient is and where they hang out.

LinkedIn

You might be wondering why we're using LinkedIn. LinkedIn is primarily used for business to business marketing. Your opportunity with regard to LinkedIn is the ability to connect with other health professionals, such as local GPs and other medics who may refer to your clinic.

A Good quality profile, republishing articles, or publishing your own articles on this platform can allow you to build a profile as the local authority in your field with other health care professionals that you wish to build a referral network with.

I use LinkedIn quite a lot with regards to my coaching business and for targeting local GPs and medics with regards to my podiatry clinic and have found it very successful for both. For an example of how to build a good quality LinkedIn profile connect with my own profile. *While there say hi and tell me how you are finding my book.*

YouTube

YouTube has over 2 billion monthly users and 30 million plus daily users. The average viewing session on YouTube is 40 minutes! With over 5 billion individual videos being watched every single day. It is the second most popular search engine globally after Google.

Using correct keywords when regards to videos you upload is important. These videos can be multi re-purposed. For example, you can embed useful videos or informational videos that you have on YouTube into your website or into your online marketing including your emails, Facebook, and so on.

Newspaper Advertising

Newspaper advertising, or magazine advertising has died away in the last few years but is still very useful with regards to local health clinics. Newspaper advertising was the first type of proper advertising I did and where I learned the importance of good copy and good message.

I have a soft spot for Newspaper advertising as it was this type of advertising that started to change my fortunes and gave me a formula to boost my new patient numbers whenever I needed to.

The three main components of a newspaper advertising is your headline, your image, the headline underneath the image and your call to action.

Again as with regards to all of your marketing when carrying out newspaper advertising you need to make sure that the ideal patient that you're targeting is reading the magazine or newspaper you're advertising in. Forgetting this basic of marketing can cost you dearly. For example, a number of years ago a local free newspaper, we regularly advertised in very successfully, ended up costing me. As I discussed earlier in this book I once decided to advertise for running injuries on a whim. We got zero responses to this, whereas in previous months, we'd had 30 to 40 responses for other conditions such as plantar fasciitis, heel pain, and so on.

I realised afterwards that the reason we had no response to the running ad was that the demographic that reads this newspaper were 60 yrs+ and were not runners and therefore not likely to have a running injury.

This does not mean that the running ad was done badly. I just had placed it in the wrong place. Had I placed it in a running magazine, we probably would have had a much greater response. In fact this is exactly what I did a number of months later, when I re-purposed the ad in a more appropriate publication.

PODIATRY BUSINESS SUCCESS SECRETS

I would urge you not to dismiss newspaper advertising. It was newspaper advertising that helped saved my business when things were looking grim.

Direct Mail.

I really love direct mail or the regular post. Yes it is old fashioned snail mail, but it is very effective when done right. Why? Well, direct mail allows you to put something physical into your prospects hands. Whether they open that letter and read it is entirely down to the quality of the advertising you do. When done right and you can certainly get their prospects to open your mail and you have their complete and utter attention.

Think about the last time you received a letter that you rushed to open before all others or a catalogue you've been waiting on. You probably poured over it and you too have the ability to do this with direct mail. You can incorporate some techniques like coloured envelopes or a handwritten address which will encourage your prospects to open your letter rather than throw it in the waste bin with all the other mass manufactured junk mail.

Often local postal service companies will offer a service where you can target your demographic quite cheaply. For example, in my area, it's possible for me for €1.00 to have my local postal service allow me design on their website a simple oversized postcard which delivers my message directly into my prospects hands in an area that I request. In some postal services this can be zeroed down to certain demographics such as family houses only, or people with a certain income level.

Oversized postcards are very successful and are quite cheap to test. I suggest first testing your copy and your headline to see what works best online such as on Facebook ads or on Google ads as this can method can give you great insights into what does and does not work at minimal cost. Once you find what's working for you, you can re-purpose this copy for direct mail, be that either letter or postcard.

As I mentioned in an earlier chapter, we use direct mail heavily in our internal marketing campaigns and have had massive responses from some multi step external and internal marketing campaigns I have utilised. For example, in my clinic we have used quite successfully (and I've had my coaching clients do the same) a 3 step direct mail campaign to local health professionals.

We begin by targeting local GPs that we want to develop a referral network with inviting them to try our services, or visit the clinic, or have us visit them to discuss how we can help their patients. Rather than having you go to every single local health Professional you hope might refer patients to you, this campaign allows them to put their hand up if they're interested and then you can work on developing that relationship.

Lumpy mail can also be incorporated into many of these campaigns to allow your campaign to stand out from all the junk mail that comes in. Lumpy mail is simply putting something physical into the letter, such as a Rubik's cube with a headline in the letter *"Puzzled about who to send your foot patients to?"* or a cheap Boomerang, which can be sent to patients who haven't come back for a while with a headline like *"We really want you back".*

If you've never heard of this type of thing before you might be thinking this is unusual. That's the whole point. There is very little new in marketing at the moment and people are bombarded with marketing throughout today and it's important that you try to make your brand and your clinic stand out from the crowd so that you have the opportunity to present your message to your potential patient or professional referral partner rather than have it muscled out by your competitors message.

Speaking At Events.

Speaking or attending events locally is a very quick and easy way to build your profile. I would ask my coaching clients to contact local groups within their area that they would like to build a referral pattern with. They may wish to build just such a relationship with their local running club so they would contact them and suggest that they do an educational talk for them.

It's important when we do these talks that we we try to continue the relationship long term, such as offering a free consult for anyone who attends the event or offer a simple discount or free screening service. Events such as a fair or summer show are a great way for you to get to target your ideal patient. Obviously, if you have no interest in helping runners for example, there will be little point in you turning up to a local 5km or 10km run. Once again you need to know your target audience and where they hang out.

Corporation free health screening is also a simple and easy way to do external marketing. Simply contact local corporations or businesses in your area and offer to come in and do a simple talk or have screening for the services that you provide.

Lastly, consider providing education to local health professionals as this can be quick and easy way to build your reputation as the local authority. I lecture every year at my local osteopathic college on foot mechanics and find that we produce a far higher turnover from the referrals we receive from those students once they qualify than I do from the payment received for that lecturing. Indeed, I've been asked many times, to give talks and lectures on various things such as marketing, coaching and podiatry itself and I'm quite happy to do so for free if appropriate as I realised that it gives me the opportunity to put myself in front of my ideal client or patient's and again build up my network of referrals.

Always be on the lookout for where you can do similar such talks in your area. While at first you may be nervous about speaking in public you need to remember two things:

No 1 .. People will take you at your own appraisal

No 2 .. Unless you push yourself outside your comfort zone you will never grow your business and you will continue to stay stuck as you are right now.

Signage Outside Your Clinic

Signage on the outside of your clinic, if you happen to have passing traffic, is a nice cheap way to drive prospects in your door. Too often I see clinics and their signage is all about themselves their qualifications and is plastered with a large logo. Your signage should be to the point and explaining the services that you provide. You could also consider having an A-Sign or similar outside your door that will allow you to change the message displayed regularly.

As an example you may offer *"Free Kids Assessments"* as when they go back to school. Change this a number of weeks later to orthotics reviews or discounted knee pain consult and so forth. I love it when my coaching clients move their clinic as it allows us to redo all of their signage and tend to find that we can boost their turnover quite quickly as a result.

Remember having attractive and more importantly effective external signage should deliver the message we want, targeting the type of patient that we want. Always follow the marketing triad.

Website.

Your website should be the hub that your entire marketing revolves around. As I said earlier, too often what happens is we develop a website having spoken to a graphic designer who really knows nothing about marketing or the psychology of the buying process but knows how to make a nice pretty website.

Your website is not there to be pretty. Your website is there to make you money. If you're in private practice and you website is not doing this or if you cannot say for certain how it makes you money then it is not designed for purpose.

My website and my coaching clients websites are primarily designed as a lead capture machine. By this I mean that we offer free information up front in exchange for our potential patients contact details, so we can follow up with them later. In the follow up or marketing funnel they are given even more useful information that answer all of their questions, overcomes all of their barriers, and ultimately leads to them choosing my clinic, or my coaching clients, clinics as the only rational choice for treatment. I firmly believe that this should be the purpose of any health professionals website.

Your clinics website purpose is not to show how great you are, what courses you've been on, and how well educated you are or how much more you care. This is the mistake that all of your competitors websites are making. Your website should be a living thing that you're constantly working on, adding and changing its content to improve its performance.

If you wish to scale your business then an effective website that encourages its visitors to take some sort of action that places them into your marketing funnels is a must. Remember, all of the external marketing and most of the internal marketing that you do will drive your patients or potential patients to your website where you want them to take the kind of action that you need, which will ultimately lead to them booking an appointment with you or your team. Any site that doesn't do this is not fit for purpose.

Chat Software On Your Website.

There are lots of different Chat/Bot software systems available, such as the one I use, *LiveChat,* that you can have on your website. This allows patients to contact your clinic by text through your website and speak to your staff without having to pick up the phone. This, while giving an impression of a more professional outfit, is particularly useful to workers in offices who don't have the ability to pick up the phone and discuss their health issues with the work colleagues overhearing.

I train my staff that once they have engaged with the prospect through the chat app that the goal is to get them on the phone as quickly as possible so we can encourage them to go ahead and make that appointment. This is a relatively cheap system, simple to set up and run and more than pays for itself over and over.

Testimonials

Depending on what part of the world you are in and depending on your society's rules you may or may not be allowed to use testimonials. If you are allowed to use testimonials, you really must do so. This will provide social proof to potential patients allowing them to see similar people to themselves that have gone through the journey in your clinic that they are considering taking. These testimonials will demonstrate outcomes others have had that have been positive and fell reassured that your clinic is the right choice.

Online testimonials are better if you can have a conversation/video with the patient and placed on your website.

These can be incorporated into the literature that you are using in your direct mail, your emails, and so forth.

When considering who to ask for testimonials, don't forget who your ideal client is and try to get testimonials from people in the same demographic. Again, if you're targeting a lady over 65 there's no point in having a testimonial of a 25 year old male triathlete. You should really try to interview a lady of the same or similar age

In Conclusion.....

As you can see, marketing is a massive topic and it's not something that we can cover in a book like this in finite detail. I will be bringing out a podiatry marketing book in the next year, so keep an eye out for us. While you wait for this, the important points I would want you to take away from this section on marketing is .....

Number 1, you must know who you're targeting.

Number 2, you must be clear on the message that you want to give them that would strike a chord with that potential patient.

Number 3, you must be clear on the media that you're going to use is the correct media, ie that your potential patient is engaging with that media.

This is why most podiatry clinics and indeed most small businesses fail at marketing. The first thing they do is they put up any sort of message on any sort of media that's offered to them. They find it gets little or no response and become frustrated with marketing and unsure of what to do next. Often this leads to them giving up marketing as not for them.

These are the kind of clinics that tell you *"I just do word of mouth marketing".*

It does not have to be like this. It is quite possible to build a marketing plan and automate it to have it running for you 24/7 allowing you to scale your business and give you the lifestyle that you require.

If this seems daunting at first don't worry. I understand this and I too felt like this when I began my journey into effective marketing.

I would urge you to start slowly, beginning with internal marketing.

Test your message, interview your potential patients to see what they're interested in and as you find out what works for you and your clinic starts to expand your marketing piece by piece.

Done right marketing has the ability to revolutionise your clinic and your life.

The secret to having a profitable and successful podiatry business with patients actively seeking your clinic out is that you need to become a great external marketer.

SECRET NO 11.

Staff, You Have To Learn To Love Them.

Whenever two or more podiatry clinic owners, or indeed two small business owners meet, the topic will often move to discussing their staff and the woes that they have with them.

There's an old clinic owners joke about how great it would be to have a clinic if it wasn't for the patients and it wasn't for the staff. While you might smile at this, the truth is without staff you the clinic owner will always have to do everything and you will never ever become truly free from the day to day grind of running a clinic. You will never ever be able to scale your clinic from a job to a true business without staff.

Instead of looking at staff as a necessary evil, I urge you to instead look at them as a vital asset you can use to build your business while delivering exceptional clinical care. You need to cherish your staff, even more so than your patients. Don't get me wrong, having staff is hard and it's sometimes extremely frustrating. A mentor of mine once told me that it was my job as clinic owner, to be as nice as possible to my staff, and to always look after them but that I should expect that "sometime one of them will s**t all over you".

My experience and taught me that this can be 100% true and I have come to appreciate that this is normal, whatever kind of business you run. You see, it used to be that as I grew my clinic I became very frustrated with my staff believing they weren't as dedicated to the clinic or as absorbed by my business as I was. However, I eventually wised up and realised that this was totally unrealistic expectation on my part.

Think about it. Your clinic is your baby. You have put your whole life into it. You have invested yourself totally into it and tied your family's well being to it.

Your staff however have other priorities;

• What's for dinner later?

• That argument with the girlfriend last night?

• Getting to the shops before they close?

• How many days until they're off and holidays?

Why would they think any other way? Your staff can walk away from your clinic and get another job at any time? Yes, it might be a bit of a hassle for them but it's much simpler for them than it would be for you to do the same thing. What you must realise as clinic owner is that this is 100% normal behaviour and you should not take personally that you and your clinic will never be your staff priority. Indeed, you should expect it.

Better to embrace the reality of the employer employee relationship.

The employer employee relationship is not an equal one. The employer has a lot of power over the employee with the ability to significantly affect their staffs lives sometimes in an arbitrary manner. Respecting this position and being seen to do so will improve your working relationship with your staff exponentially.

Too often I see a poor, even toxic, atmosphere in clinics with the owner and staff almost acting as adversaries instead of as team players. While the clinic owner will often blame the staff for a poor atmosphere, ultimately how your staff perform and the atmosphere in the clinic is directly related to what you the clinical owner tolerates.

You would get the staff you deserve.

I have had lots of various problems and stresses with staff over the years and when I look back, almost all of it was avoidable and 99% of it was my fault. It was my fault for allowing the culture of the clinic to be such that I, on occasion, used to sit in my car outside my own business, just talking myself into going in to the clinic to work with staff and an atmosphere that was raising my stress levels daily.

The Culture Of Your Business

Just ask my wife and she will tell you that I am not sentimentalist, into feng shui or centring my zen. She says that I am a transactionalist and she is probably right as she is in most things. While the term culture in business is bandied around in an often phoney way with little action to back it up, I am a firm believer in having a positive and vibrant culture in your clinic.

It is possible to determine and structure the culture of your business as you wish.

To me culture means the ethos of how you want your business to function every day in every way. All businesses have a culture even if they have never actually considered this to be the case.

When I had first began to scale my clinic, without really knowing what I was doing, I had a pretty crappy culture. It was a work environment where staff are unsure of their requirements by the owner, me, who was also not clear on what he was doing or where he was trying to get to. Some days, you could cut the tension in the clinic with a knife. For a small practice with a small team, this was not a pleasant place to come to work for any of us. Internally, I accepted that the fault was mine, and I set out to make a change.

How To Design Your Clinics Culture

To begin with, I took time away from work to consider my goals and by extension, the goals of the clinic. I realised my ultimate goal was to achieve freedom. Freedom to choose what kind of work I did. Freedom to go to work on almost any given day if I decided I wanted to.

I wanted a business that would be able to provide a modest lifestyle for my family, without the constant financial worries that most Podiatry clinic owners seem to have and to provide financial security for my family in the long term, not just make a quick buck.

I have pretty modest tastes and have no interest in a lavish lifestyle and I believe that most podiatry clinic owners are the same. They're looking to deliver best quality medical care in an ethical fashion by providing enough profit to justify the extra responsibility and stresses that come with running that business and having staff.

To achieve my goals, I needed to build a business that was independent of me while also providing my family and I with the freedom we desired. I needed a clinic that provided the best possible podiatry medical care as an essential. By putting my staff and my patients first, front and centre then they would in turn provide me with what I needed, while also ensuring the business delivered for all of its stakeholders, its staff, its patients and its suppliers.

The Steps I Took to Re-frame My Clinics Poor Culture

Step 1. I wanted to be able to write in one single sentence what the goal of my clinic was, should anybody asked. I decided what I wanted to achieve for my clinic was

"To help people live their best lives by keeping them Active and Mobile in a holistic way that recognises them as a person first a patient second."

Step 2. I set out to create a short number of core values that are wanted my clinic to demonstrate daily and expand on them. The expectation was that this would in turn lead to our purpose being fulfilled. All of this so far would be for the public/patients consumption and was to be placed prominently within the clinic and on its website.

Step 3. I closed the clinic for half a day, locked the doors, unplugged the phones and bought a big tray of donuts for all of the staff. I started this half day by opening the meeting explaining what it was I wanted to achieve from the meeting and apologised for any part that I personally had in any negativity in the clinic in the past. I took full responsibility for the past and present atmosphere in the clinic ie; its culture and that the buck would always stop with me.

I went on then to detail my vision for the clinic and the importance I felt that we were all 100% clear on our core values, our purpose and our culture. I admitted that I had naively assumed that all staff shared my value system with regards to work.

This would happen no more and that I was sharing these core values and purpose with them and placing them in a public place within the clinic to act as a reminder to ourselves and as a commitment to each other and our patients and other stakeholders of how we will interact even in times of stress.

We went on to discuss these core values and their meaning and situations where we would have to live by them in work. Having completed this section on core values over a number of hours, I then set about devising a set of loose rules and enforcement's which were devised and agreed upon by the staff, not me.

My role was simply to enable them to do so and to make sure that they would have the understanding that all staff including me would follow them in our day to day dealings with each other.

By allowing the staff working for my clinic on that day to set our belief system they would hopefully gain ownership of this and by extension the culture of the clinic and its continuing maintenance. To truly work as a successful team these needed to be a set of rules, a set of simple but powerful rules that govern the internal behaviour of any team, organisation etc.

These rules while not for public consumption would become the heart of the team and when combined with the core values, our vision and purpose I the founder had for the clinic, it would become our culture, which we would all invest in and protect.

While the company already had legal contracts and legal employee handbooks, these more personal statements allowed a culture of mutual support and understanding to develop with a set of standards of conduct and performance which were upheld.

All new staff that joined the team subsequent to this entered a work environment whereby before they even started working they were instructed and initiated on our culture, our core values and our belief system and that they would need to accept it as the way it was done in our clinic before they joined. Indeed, they were told that if they had an issue and couldn't live by these rules, this culture, they should not take the position.

Older staff demonstrated by their words and their actions that this was non negotiable, nor was it subject to interpretations, but that in times of stress or confusion could be relied upon for guidance and support. The supportive culture has led to a happier atmosphere for all whereby working as a team we all succeed. The clinic does not rely on the owner having to decide or enforce the rules as we as a group support each other or call each other out when needed.

At this point an undertaking, that I was worried was going to lead to me looking like a fool at best or losing control of work, has in fact led to a more trustworthy cohesion and energy in the team, a team that is self reliant and embedded in each team member is our purpose and values.

The culture of the clinic now is the best I have ever worked in in all of my years and is driven not by me, but by the staff themselves.

For a lot of clinic owners who have for so long ploughed their own furrow the idea of giving up control to their staff on how their clinic reaches its purpose is a huge leap of faith. However, I strongly believe that it's a leap worth taking and even if it's just you on your own in that clinic, I urge you to go through this process, perhaps sitting down with a significant other to do so.

Set the foundation now, for a positive and prescribed culture and you will take a huge step towards a truly successful clinic. Any new staff that may join you in future will be absorbed into this culture ensuring a smoother and more pleasant work environment for all.

Two books, I would urge you to consider getting your hands on that I found extremely useful while undergoing this enterprise were

"Culture Is Everything" by Tristan White & *"Team Code Of Honor"* by Blair Singer.

You will also find a copy of clinics, Core Values & Belief System at this books bonus page exclusively for readers of this book and members of my coaching programme...

www.morepracticeprofits.com/podiatry-business-book-bonus

Hiring.

So if you are in the lucky position today of needing or wanting to take on another team member you really will need to have a plan. Instead usually what happens is that when the clinic owner decides they want someone they have a look online at what their competitors are doing, copy their ad for the job even if it's not very effective and throw up a similar advertisement online or on their professional societies Facebook group or in their publication.

This is a recipe for disaster. If you have no plan on how you will go about recruitment and your marketing for new staff members is substandard the type of applications that you receive will also be substandard.

You need to have a plan just like you do when trying to attract new patients.

- **You need to consider firstly, who it is you want to attract.**

- **What type of clinician or admin team member do you want?**

- **What tasks or roles will they have and what traits or characteristics will they need to have in abundance to do the job?**

People often say go for personality, but really what they mean is go for the character or characteristics that will allow them to excel in the position you have available.

Once you've done this first but crucial step, then consider what does this type of person want from a job? Is it all about money, is it education, is it flexibility and working hours and so forth. When you know who you want to attract and you know what they want, only then do you design your message around that and place the advertisement where they will see it.

Remember the Marketing Triad.

When you have your applications and you move on to your interview, you need to make sure that the questions you have are designed to find out whether or not the candidates have the characteristics needed to fulfill the role you have available. Questions like "What are your strengths and weaknesses?" or other stereotypical questions are not going to give you the knowledge you need to make an educated decision on who is the right candidate for the position.

I always like to have a non clinician sit in with me as they would have a very different perspective to me. Clinicians or other podiatrists like myself will tend to focus on the candidates education, their qualifications and their clinical skills almost at the expense of all else. What good is a staff member with a PhD if they can't look your patient in the eye, if they can't empathize with them, or can't get that patient to agree to the treatment plan required to ensure the patient reaches their goal .

Personally, I'm not looking for the best CV, or the most experience. I have tended to find that the best staff members to take on have always been new grads, as they have little or no preconceptions on how the job should be done. This allows me to mould them to work the way I want them to, using our systems.

I'm looking for characteristics such as the ability to follow my systems or willingness to learn, a willingness to be a team player and the ability to follow our core values and to buy into them. Indeed, in the interview process, we go through our core values. We explain the importance of them and if we feel that this interviewee is not going to meet our core values, they proceed no further.

PODIATRY BUSINESS SUCCESS SECRETS

Once you have a shortlist of possible candidates, I suggest making a list of the top four or five traits or characteristics that you need and you score them out of for example, 10. Add up the scores and get a score out of 40 or 50. Now, it's not necessarily that you need to give the job to whoever gets the greatest score, but this does give you some more information and will often help to confirm your impression from the interview.

Again, this is best not done on your own but rather with another member of staff who was in the interview process.

When you have chosen your candidate and you are ready to meet them you will do so to negotiate. This is a very important meeting as you need to do two things in this meeting; sell them the job and set the parameters or expectations of the person who fills the position. Remember to use the candidates emotional goal to get them to buy into your position. They will rationalise it later.

Make sure to be 100% clear on the expectations that you have for them in that position. Be as detailed as you can, so that there's no misconceptions when they start a job, or six months or 12 months later on what you meant by what you needed them to do.

Don't be in a rush to pick anybody. The worst thing to do will be to pick someone just because they're available. Better to wait for the right person than the wrong person in the wrong position and have to remove them eventually. I have learned this the hard way and now I'm happy to wait months if needed to get the right person.

Once you have agreed to take them on and they have agreed to the parameters/expectations and are happy to be held accountable you can shake hands and move on to the next step.

Keeping Your Staff

The way the world economy and labour markets have evolved staff, especially younger staff, tend to move on after a number of years. There's no such thing has a job for life anymore and if you expect that your staff are going to stay with you forever you're being completely unrealistic.

Sometimes in an effort to stop their staff from leaving, clinic owners make foolish decisions such as partnerships, selling part of their business too soon, etc.

The clinic owners job is to make their staff replaceable while the staffs job is to make themselves irreplaceable. In a work environment like we have now where there is a shortage of allied health professionals, it is in the clinic owners interest to try and hold on that staff member as long as possible considering the effort that's been put into recruiting and training them. Whatever you do, do not over promise as it may be something you live to regret.

Money may not be the driving factor for your staff and if it is, perhaps that is not the right staff member for you, as they may never be satisfied. It's more likely with the type of workforce that is coming out of college now that they have a need for a feeling of self worth and progression within their career. Indeed, recent research shows that staff who have a feeling such as this or sense that they are contributing are happier in a job and will tend to stay longer than those who are simply paid more. You need to have a system to make sure that this happens, that your staff are happy and feel fulfilled at work.

In my coaching program, I help my clients to devise a retention system for their staff just like I have done in my clinic. I do quite a number of things to encourage my staff to stay. These include having a CPD fund that's there for them to spend on courses they wish to do. We have active training and mentorship programs in place whereby junior staff are taken under the wing of more senior staff member and helped progress. We have regular social occasions paid for by the clinic which is devised for team building and rapport. The clinic will invest in and encourage them to develop their long term future and happiness and let them know that this is a priority of the clinic. Indeed this is encapsulated in our Core Values.

One of the biggest issues that leads to employer-employee breakdown is the lack of clearly defined goals or what is expected of the employee by the employer. These expectations of each other is often left unsaid or assumed by the employer and the employee.

This can be easily resolved before the employee takes the job by having;

Number 1; Clear objective goals such as percentage of patients that complete their plan of care, good quality medical records kept and so on

Number 2; Continual accountability of these goals and meetings to assess the performance of that employee.

Number 3; Any issues that need to be dealt with should be done so in an environment of positivity and continual, individual and group improvement.

Again all of this goes back to our core values and that these core values are continually upheld by the employer and the employee. If you have clear understandable systems, an energetic mentorship and CPD program and clear goals are assessed objectively your staff will be happier and feel more secure in their position. As a result of this they will tend to stay with you for longer and recommend you to their peers as the place to come and work.

Should I take on a receptionist or another podiatrist?

One of the top questions asked by clinic owners considering scaling up is whether they should take on another Podiatrist or employ a receptionist first.

A lot of clinic owners assume that the first thing they should do is take on another podiatrist when they are ready to scale. Often these clinic owners mistakenly feel that a receptionist is not contributing financially to the clinic and that instead of podiatrist who can charge for the patient's they will see will be bringing in far more money than any receptionist could.

I can see what their argument. It is very easy to see what a new podiatrist is bringing in per hour but it is much more difficult to do the same with a receptionist.

However, this is where we disagree. I have always found that a well trained front desk staff member is far harder for re-place and will boost your turnover, enhance profitability and reduce your stress levels as the clinic owner far far more than any podiatrist will.

A good quality receptionist or front desk staff member will do a number of things for you if train them well. They will interact with the public before they become a patient and depending on the conversation will determine whether or not that potential patient will turn in to a happy customer of yours.

They will be able to enact any follow up procedures you have that need to happen with leads that are generated from your marketing plan. In fact they should be able to implement the majority of your marketing plan you devised allowing you free to carry out more profitable and higher level tasks. These tasks may be treating patient's or devising more marketing campaigns or simply having the time and energy to focus on scaling your podiatry clinic into a true business.

A valuable admin member will be able to take over most if not all of your admin duties, leaving you the owner less stressed giving you the freedom to choose whether to or not to attend your clinic all of the time, yet still be open, still taking bookings and still bringing in income. No podiatrists with the focus on treating patients will be able to do these things.

I always suggest to any sole practitioners considering what to do that it's better to take on a front desk or receptionist before taking on your first podiatrist, even if you can only do so part time.

Once you take on your receptionist, have them well trained, they will be a marketing machine for you turning leads into patients and boosting your turnover. This will allow you to then take on a podiatrist whose book will be filled much much faster than it would otherwise and allow you the ability to continue the process scaling as you go.

PODIATRY BUSINESS SUCCESS SECRETS

Lastly, a well trained front desk staff member will be able to fill the book of more than one podiatrists that work for you should you wish, where as a new podiatrist can really only fill their own book.

So before you consider taking on another podiatrist, perhaps you should consider scaling up your administration team first.

Firing Staff

Firing staff is an unfortunate part of running a health business that all employers must get used to no matter how much you want to avoid it. The last thing you want to do is to have a staff member that is not performing remain in their position even after all options have been exhausted to improve that. In many a clinic, the employer avoids firing staff as it is too uncomfortable and over time the atmosphere turns toxic.

"Fire Fast & Hire Slow" is a commonly used and appropriate saying in business and one you should adopt.

If your staff member is not working out and you've tried everything you could to resolve the situation then make sure that they are removed as quickly as possible, making sure before you begin this process at all, that you have solid legal advice behind you. I suggest to my clients that they get expert

HR help at all stages. When it comes to dealing with staff we are not HR experts, nor should we try to be.

Similarly, when it comes to contracts, we should be getting expert help. I have seen clinic owners try to save a few pounds by doing the contract themselves, something they found on the internet or a simple shake of the hand. This is a recipe for disaster, as there is no legal document to revert to, should any disagreements occur and in the long term cost of clinic owner far more than they would have ever paid out had they invested in the right advice on day one.

Indeed in most podiatry clinics the staff are self employed rather than an employee. I have done this in the past and would argue that if this arrangement can be avoided it should be. I understand the perceived benefits of your staff being self-employed are to the clinic owner. The clinic owner doesn't have to concern themselves with the staff members tax and there's less man management.

However, an employee will be easier to manage and will be more pliable to adaptation to your changing circumstances than any self employed member of your team. This is vital if you're planning to scale as things will definitely change.

Likewise, paying a staff member a percentage of their turnover means they're far less likely to agree to any changes including those that will occur associated with trying to systemise or scale your business. They will view the probability that it could lead to a potential loss of income in the short or medium term for that self employed person.

I found through bitter experience that it is better to pay a guaranteed wage which will allow you to maximise productivity and turnover alike while scaling and also allow your staff member to feel secure as these changes occur.

The key to having a good staffing relationship is

1. **Have a healthy and live culture in your clinic.**

2. **Be mindful of the unequal employer-employee relationship.**

3. **Have empathy for your staff.**

4. **Be clear on the role and expectations that you have of your staff.**

5. **Have frequent meetings with those staff with objective performance reviews.**

6. **Have an active educational element to their position with active support from the clinic.**

7. **Avoid micromanagement or personalising any situation.**

Train, trust, measure, repeat.

Having staff can be hard. Sometimes it's like having kids except you can't send them to your room, but if you manage it well, you are respectful of them and you hold them accountable to their performance they will provide you with the lifestyle that you desire while also being able to provide your patients with the best quality medical care.

The secret to having a great podiatry clinic is to cherish your staff and accept the stresses that come with being the boss, but realise that having staff is the key to scaling a successful and profitable Podiatry clinic.

You simply cannot do it alone.

SECRET NO 12.

How do I scale my podiatry clinic?

Firstly, for those of you asking *"Why should I scale my podiatry clinic?"* I realise that having staff or going beyond just yourself is not what everybody reading this book wants and that's perfectly fine with me.

Some want to avoid the stress of staff, building their clinic up from beyond just simply a job to business. That does not mean that this Secret is not for you. At some point you may wish to sell on your clinic and if you have systematised your business it will make it easier to sell and more profitable when you do so.

The easier it is to replace yourself, the easier it will be to have someone else slip into your position when you are ready to move on. A huge mistake I see a lot of clinic owners making is trying to build a business that depends solely on them. They are needed for all sorts of decisions, even the small ones. Decisions such as ordering, paying bills, doing the marketing (if any), treating the patients of course, bookkeeping and so on.

Let's be honest, most Podiatry clinics are just like this, where the principal podiatrist is depended on for pretty much everything. The owner provides most of the turnover and no decision is made without them. No matter how many staff you have, this is not a true business, but rather a highly paid job.

A lot of podiatry clinic owners never let go of the reins of their business. They never allow the staff to be able to make any decisions and are poor at delegating. This means that they are tied to the business. These clinic owners find it difficult to switch off and have difficulty taking any leave as they are constantly worried about decisions that are being made in their absence and the loss of revenue from their not seeing patients. These podiatry clinic owners are never able to move on from working "in their business" to working "on their business". I too was just like this.

Scaling your clinic even if it's just you, at this point will help to allow you the business owner to free yourself from the daily grind of having to make every decision and be there all of the time. Using the following processes I've been able to scale my Podiatry clinic by 400%, increase my profits by over 400% and still growing, take holidays away from work for up to four weeks at a time and come back to a business that runs efficiently without me.

We medical clinicians tend to be perfectionists. After all, we cannot afford to be slipshod with our medical care. It is drummed into us in university that we must be almost infallible. It is because of this that we tend to, as a group, be almost glacial in letting go of the reins of the clinic and trusting others with tasks that up until then we have performed.

I know of podiatry clinics that, even after 25 years of being open, the principal podiatrist and founder still refuses to let anyone else do biomechanics orthotics and so on *"because they may not do it my way"*. These clinics are really just a highly paid high pressure job which will be very hard to sell on come retirement, as the principal *is* the business. These tend to be the kind of clinics that new staff join full of enthusiasm and after a number of years know that they're having no opportunity to develop their skills, as the owner is unwilling to let them perform tasks that they prefer to do. These staff members tend to move on and in a lot of cases, open a clinic quite close by.

The key to earning more, working less, living the life you truly want and having an asset that you can then sell on when you are ready is the following 5 simple steps;

1. **Develop systems for everything in your clinic**

2. **Train staff on those systems**

3. **Delegate to those staff using the systems they are trained on**

4. **Review performance regularly with clearly defined goals**

5. **Repeat steps 1 to 4 and scale up**

1. Developing Systems.

Whenever I begin working with a client in my coaching business and I ask them to tell me about their systems, they usually tell me that they don't have any. This is simply not true. Normally, they have some sort of systems, they just so happen to not be very good systems and to have put little or no thought into recording those systems.

Every podiatry clinic, indeed every small business has a way of doing things. The way to answer the phone, a way to take payments, the way to open or close the clinic and so on. However, for most of these clinics the systems are informal systems or they just happened to be the way that it's done in that clinic. They are systems that have just developed organically over time.

To begin to develop your systems simply start by making a record of the way that you want things done as the clinic owner if you were not there. This can be done by a number of ways, including video, simple text, audio, screen recording of PowerPoint presentation etc. It should be a simple step by step set of instructions on how to do a certain task. The less complex it is, the better. The point is, once you have it stored, you have a system.

Of course it's natural that once you have started developing these systems you'll want to tweak them and improve them as time goes by. Just because you have a system does not mean that you can't improve or make changes. Not only can you alter your systems but you should be constantly doing so as you find newer and better ways of doing the things that need to be done.

Now to systemise your clinic is a big job and to be honest, will never be fully finished. But don't let this put you off beginning. Just make a start and keep going. If you do only one system a day, five days a week, that's 250 odd systems in a year. One of my favourite sayings is "How do you eat an elephant?..... One bite at a time."

Personally, I like to have a combination of video screen recording and typed up systems all kept in the cloud in a systems manual, such as Google Drive which you can acquire for free. This way it can be accessed by any member of staff at the click of a button.

2. Train Staff On Those Systems.

As you develop your systems, you will need to train your staff on them making sure to not make this process complicated. Simply give them access to the system. I like to send my staff the system before organising regular meetings to go over the training or system and answer any questions my staff may have.

As you repeat this process over and over, you will refine how you'd like to train your staff.

3. Delegate To Your Staff

The whole purpose of this systematisation of your business is that your staff will end up doing the things that you the owner needs them to do in the way that you want them to do it.

A simple tip is to make sure that your system is simple enough to be understood by a 10 year old. I have four small kids at the time I'm writing this, my eldest being 10 years of age. He's always coming into the clinic stealing all of the biscuits and all of my staff know him well. When I've asked them to write a system for me, I tell them to write it as if they're writing it for him. This means the system will be simple enough that any member of staff that joins in the future will be able to understand.

3.1 What Does It Mean To Delegate To Those Trained Staff?

When I say delegate, I do not mean abdicate. As owner, you cannot say to your staff... *"You know what I want done, now don't bother me again"*. Yes, you must trust them but remember, you need to delegate to scale, but never abdicate. A bonus to this delegation can also include having your staff developing those systems and training future staff.

In my clinic, I have had more senior members of my staff develop an automated 16 week training system for new podiatrists that would join the clinic. The same senior staff members also as well as developing this system train the newer members on it meaning I no longer have to develop the system anymore. Nor do I have to provide all the training, freeing me up to do other tasks such a writing this book!

4. Review Performance.

Making sure that you are regularly reviewing your staffs performance is vital to the smooth scaling up of your clinic. Regular meetings, both in groups and one to one, whereby you hold your staff accountable and assess if your systems are being followed will lead to your staff realising that it's your clinic systems way or no way.

It would not be unusual for newer staff members to have 1 to 2 or sometimes even 3 meetings per week with a more senior member of staff for training and checking that they're following our processes and systems.

While you might be thinking this is lost patient hours and income, in the long run, what this leads to is having a growing number staff doing it your way without you having to be there. When a system is not being followed be sure to correct this and if it becomes a continual issue with an individual, take the appropriate steps to rectify this, making sure that you are getting HR/legal advice if appropriate.

There is a fine line between being too lenient and micromanaging but the great thing about being the boss is that you are in charge and you get to say how things should be done.

I remember the last time I went away for a month and the day I returned to work we had a two hour meeting of all staff as we do every single week. I asked what issues have arisen over the month and only two or three issues needed to be brought to my attention. When I asked the whole team why they had happened and ultimately what was done wrong their answer to me was, *"we didn't follow the system"*.

This was wonderful to see, as it showed that the staff had bought into the idea of following the system because it was designed to help them not hinder them.

5. Repeat & Scale

By repeating this process over and over, you will begin to free yourself and move more and more tasks from your to do list to your staffs so that you can focus on higher and more profitable tasks such as mentoring your staff or internal and external marketing.

By following exactly this process, I have been able to scale my podiatry clinic over 400% and still growing, reduce my clinical hours to an average of 5 per week and give me time to open my podiatry coaching business helping other podiatry clinic owners make the most of their businesses.

Systematising your podiatry clinic will result in uniformity in the completion of the tasks that up until then you are doing in your clinic. This includes all aspects of operations from stocktaking to answering the phone. Even systematising to the level of the shape of the padding that you want applied to patient's feet will lead to your patients having an almost exact same experience no matter who they meet within your clinic.

This will result in allowing you to begin to scale while still delivering the same standard of customer care and medical treatment that would occur had you seen every single patient.

It will also mean that any staff leaving will be less of a drama than it is in most clinics as it is the system that determines what happens, not that particular individual team member and you the owner will have predetermined what that system will be. These things will be done your way even when you are not there, no matter who the staff member is.

Areas you should consider systematising in no particular order include ;

• Administration,

• Finances,

• Non clinician patient contacts such as new patient welcoming

• Marketing both internal and external

• Clinical treatment planning

- Day to day clinic running such as opening or closing up

- HR system

- Health and Safety

- Patient note taking

- Staff Training

- CPD

- Performance review meeting

The secret to having a podiatry clinic that runs the way you want even if you are not there is to have detailed systems, training and trusting your staff.

This will give you the freedom to allow you to begin to scale your clinic into a true business that will provide you with the opportunity to Earn More, Work Less and Live The Life You Desire.

SECRET NO 13.

Get A Podiatry Business Coach.

Congratulations, you have got all the way to the end and I hope by this stage are brimming with enthusiasm to begin to make the changes needed to your podiatry clinic to ensure it reaches its maximum potential.

I know you might be asking why I gave away so many of the secrets I used in my clinic. I was asked why I don't just keep it all for members of my coaching programme?

The truth is most podiatrists who read this book will never meet me, or attend one of my online or in-person courses or buy one of the products on my website.

I understand that, but does not mean I cannot help them achieve more with their clinic. I don't believe that Podiatry should be a profession where you have to struggle if you decide to go into private practice. I want my fellow podiatrists to have a rewarding career.

What I really wish from this book is to reach that clinic owner who is the same position I was in a few years ago. Tied to their clinic, working harder than ever and not seeing the benefits they hoped for. Perhaps just like I was they are living from week to week, never able to take a long holiday as they needed to keep the wheels turning.

If just one podiatry clinic owner who is at the end of their rope and feeling overwhelmed reads this book and it helps to open their eyes and see that there is another way then I will be satisfied.

It is possible to have a clinic that delivers ethical best practice medical care and deliver to you the owner the lifestyle you yearn. It is possible to earn more while working less yet giving even better quality customer service to even more people.

This is what I help my coaching clients achieve in my business More Practice Profits. I started More Practice Profits to help clinic owners like you. I have lived the life of a stressed out overworked, underpaid clinic owner. I know what it's like to feel like you are working all the time but making no money, no progress and wonder why you ever started your own clinic.

I passionately believe that it is possible to deliver exceptional customer service,best practice patient care and still deliver a fantastic lifestyle for the clinic owner.

By helping clinic owners to implement internal management, marketing & conversion systems I wanted to help

Health Business owners build a real business that allows them the life they dreamed of when they opened their doors for the first time.

—◁○▷—

Clients like Mark & Stephen Ryan podiatry clinic owners at Foot Focus, Dublin, Ireland;

Working with Lorcan has been a great experience for us and our clinic. Before we started working with him we were very focused on being busy. We had reached the point where we were very busy treating patients during normal office hours. However we had no time to manage other areas of the business.

Lorcan has helped us greatly in differentiating between having a job and having a business. Through working with Lorcan we have realised the importance of taking a step back from treating patients constantly to looking at the business as a whole and taking in the broader picture. Initially it was quite overwhelming but through implementing Lorcan's suggested systems and standardising procedures across our clinics it has helped us to be more organised and increased our productivity.

I would highly recommend working with Lorcan if you want to make the most out of the hours you put in rather than constantly feeling under pressure and overwhelmed.

Or Peter Gauntlett podiatry clinic owner at Lewisham Foot Health, London.

When I first started working with Lorcan I was feeling that my practice was running me. I was unable to take charge and make the decisions needed to move my practice forward to the next level. As a podiatrist, my main interest was in treating and getting people better. I had failed to see the opportunities that a podiatry business can offer me.

As we started working together, Lorcan gave me the confidence to value my work and help set in motion the systems needed to build a practice that reflected the hard work I had already invested. He supports and encourages and understands how to get you to a mindset where you can start building the systems and professional approach to cope with the changes that need to be implemented to move forward.

He is a good listener and knows how to get to the core of the matter in a sensitive and professional way. He has a lot of insight into how people think and behave and because he has built his own business he knows what you are going through.

His no nonsense approach made me trust him immediately and his direct style of coaching makes it easy to understand the steps you should take to improve your practice and increase your profits.

Lorcan being a successful multi-practice owner with over 20 years of experience of being in business has the know-how and expertise to move you forward to create the practice you had dreamed about.

If you are looking for a business mentor – coach then I can't recommend Lorcan highly enough.

I can help you reach your business and life goals faster and avoid the mistakes that can lead to having a business that fails to deliver the lifestyle you want.

Let me help you deliver a health business that works without you, just like I have done, while at the same time increasing your income, building better systems, marketing and delivering Wow customer service levels.

Together we can define your goals and reach them faster, allowing you to spend more time with the people your love.

Whether we ever work together or not I urge you to remember that you are not alone in business. There is help out there for you. You just have to ask for it.

Good luck in all of you endeavours.

Lorcan O Donaile, Podiatrist & Health Business Mentor.

More Practice Profits.

Remember to get your Free Bonus Materials available to readers of this book at

www.morepracticeprofits.com/podiatry-business-book-bonus

ABOUT THE AUTHOR

Lorcan O'Donaile is an Irish Podiatrist and Health Business Mentor.

He qualified from London Foot Hospital & University College London in 1998 and moved into private practice opening his own clinic, Achilles Foot Clinic, Cork, Ireland in 2005. In 2012 he expanded to open Keep Active Physio.

He guest lectures on Podiatry in Ireland and the business of Podiatry.

Having made every possible mistake you can in running your own clinic he has gone on to study and apply business principles to his clinic.

His clinic now runs as an automated business generating the profits that give him the freedom to decide if he will consult with patients or take time off to spend with his wife and small children.

This freedom has allowed him to develop his other passion... helping other clinic owners to Earn More, Work Less & Enjoy Their Life.

DOWNLOAD THE BONUSES AVAILABLE FOR READERS OF THIS BOOK FOR FREE AT ......

www.morepracticeprofits.com/podiatry-business-book-bonus

Printed in Poland
by Amazon Fulfillment
Poland Sp. z o.o., Wrocław